Skin Deep:

The History, Harm, and Healing of Modern Beauty

Copyright and Legal Disclaimer

© 2025 Jenece Mordt M.Ed. All rights reserved.

No part of this publication may be reproduced, stored in a retrieval system, or transmitted in any form or by any means—electronic, mechanical, photocopying, recording, or otherwise—without the prior written permission of the author, except in the case of brief quotations embodied in critical articles or reviews.

This book is intended for informational and educational purposes only. It is not intended to serve as medical or psychological advice, diagnosis, or treatment. The information presented in *Skin Deep* reflects the author's personal experience, research, and interpretation of available scientific literature and ancestral practices. Readers should consult with a qualified healthcare professional before making any changes to their diet, lifestyle, or skincare routine.

The author and publisher disclaim any liability for any adverse effects resulting from the use of the information contained in this book.

Product names, trademarks, and brands mentioned are the property of their respective owners and do not imply endorsement.

For permissions, interviews, or rights inquiries, contact: carnivoregrannychats@gmail.com

INTRODUCTION:	4
Mirror, Mirror... Who Told You That Was Beautiful?	4
CHAPTER 1:	7
Paint, Poison & Powder: A Timeline of Dangerous Beauty	7
CHAPTER 2:	18
The Invention of Flaws	18
CHAPTER 3:	24
Beautifully Unregulated	24
CHAPTER 4:	37
Hormones Hijacked	37
CHAPTER 5:	48
Skin Deep Symptoms	48
CHAPTER 6:	57
The "Natural" Lie	57
CHAPTER 7:	67
The Mirror Mindset Detox	67
CHAPTER 8:	79
The Beauty Rebellion	79
CHAPTER 9:	88
Building Your Clean Living Toolkit	88
CHAPTER 10:	98
Community, Culture & Conversation	98
CHAPTER 11:	105
Staying Rooted	105
CHAPTER 12:	115
What Beauty Really Is	115
APPENDIX:	122
Tools for the Journey	122

INTRODUCTION:

Mirror, Mirror... Who Told You That Was Beautiful?

You remember your first lipstick, don't you? Maybe it was a dusty rose, maybe fire engine red. It felt like a rite of passage. You stood in the mirror, twisted the tube, and became someone new. You were told it made you pretty. You were told it made you *more*. And if you're like most of us, you never questioned what was in it. Not then, and maybe not even now.

For decades, we've been seduced by glossy magazine pages, billion-dollar marketing campaigns, and passed-down rituals that whisper, shout, and sometimes scream that beauty equals worth. We've smeared lead across our eyelids, sprayed plastic onto our hair, and rubbed hormone-disrupting chemicals directly into the largest organ of our body, our skin. All in the name of being "presentable," "feminine," or simply "enough."

But beauty was never supposed to be a war. Not against your age. Not against your pores. And certainly not against your health. Yet here we are, exhausted, inflamed, and buried under layers of lotions and lies.

This book is a call to wake up. To look behind the shimmer and glow. To understand what we've really been sold. Because when we talk about beauty, we are also talking about illness, fertility, identity, control, and profit. Beauty isn't just about how you look. It's about how you live, and how you're manipulated into living a certain way.

We are going to dig up the roots. The old ones soaked in lead, arsenic, and radium. We're going to examine how ancient rituals got twisted into billion-dollar industries. We are going to pull apart the silent deals between regulators and corporations, and expose the myth that modern science has made beauty safer. And then, we're going to rebuild. From the ground up. With tallow, salt, earth, and the kind of truth that doesn't come in a bottle.

You're not broken. You never were. But the system that told you otherwise is.

We don't need another serum. We need a revolution.

Let's begin with a journey through time, peeling back the centuries to uncover the toxic legacy of beauty, starting with the earliest civilizations and working forward to the toxic aisles of today.

CHAPTER 1:

Paint, Poison & Powder: A Timeline of Dangerous Beauty

Before there was Sephora, there were salt mines and ash. Before "clean beauty" became a marketing tool, true beauty rituals were rooted in the earth. Women used clay, tallow, fermented herbs, and sunlight. Beauty was a practice tied to health, to seasons, to soil. But somewhere along the way, paint turned to poison, and ritual turned to revenue. It did not happen overnight. It crept in like lead through a lipstick tube.

Ancient Egypt: Lead and Legacy

When we think of ancient Egypt, we picture gold, opulence, and striking beauty. Cleopatra, draped in linen and jewels, is often idolized as the original queen of glam. Her image is iconic, but beneath that beauty lay layers of danger. The dramatic, smoky eye that defined Egyptian allure was created using kohl, a cosmetic made from ground galena, or lead sulfide. It gave depth to the eyes, protected against the sun's glare, and was even believed to ward off evil spirits. But what it also did, silently and relentlessly, was poison the bloodstream (Goldwater, 1972).

Lead, once absorbed through the thin skin around the eyes, travels throughout the body. It accumulates in tissues, interferes with neurological function, and affects reproductive health. The Egyptians didn't know the full extent of the damage, but they did notice its effects: fatigue, tremors, miscarriages. Still, these symptoms were tolerated, even expected, among the elite. Appearance overruled health. This is a pattern that has repeated itself in nearly every era of cosmetic history.

Make no mistake: beauty in ancient Egypt was spiritual, cultural, and deeply personal. But it was also political. Cleopatra's makeup wasn't just vanity. It was power, projection, and perception. By painting her eyes in toxic minerals, she wielded influence, asserted dominance, and adhered to her society's most sacred beauty rituals. These rituals were steeped in belief, but also in blindness.

It wasn't only Cleopatra. Lower-class Egyptian women used similar kohl mixtures, often in higher concentrations. Children had their eyes rimmed in black before they could even walk. Entire generations were exposed to toxic metals daily in the name of protection, health, and beauty. And while kohl may have had some antibacterial properties, the lead content far outweighed the benefit (Shah et al., 2016).

Why does this matter now? Because we are still doing it. We are still accepting harmful ingredients in our pursuit of an ideal. An ideal passed down from a lineage of painted faces and poisoned bloodstreams. The legacy of ancient Egypt isn't just in pyramids and hieroglyphs. It is in our medicine cabinets, our makeup bags, and our unexamined beliefs about what makes us beautiful.

The Roman Empire: Mercury and Madness

The Roman Empire was a society obsessed with appearances-particularly skin. Pale, smooth complexions were more than just aesthetic ideals; they were symbols of privilege, cleanliness, and elite status. Tanned or weathered skin was associated with labor and poverty, while light, unblemished skin communicated a life of luxury, wealth, and access.

To achieve this ethereal look, Roman elites-both men and women-turned to dangerous skin-whitening products. Chief among them were mercury-based creams. These concoctions, often made with mercuric chloride or calomel (a mercury compound), were applied daily in an effort to bleach the skin. While they initially gave the illusion of porcelain purity, they came at a steep cost.

Mercury is a potent neurotoxin. Prolonged use of these creams led to a host of severe health problems: memory loss, tremors, anxiety, insomnia, reproductive issues, and in more advanced cases, hallucinations and madness. The symptoms were slow to manifest, often misattributed to other causes, and tragically accepted as the price of beauty. Roman physicians documented these effects, but the knowledge was not enough to curb the trend.

What made these practices even more insidious was their normalization across gender lines. Unlike many ancient cultures, Roman society permitted (and even encouraged) men to participate in beauty rituals. Wealthy men would visit bathhouses and apply the same whitening creams and rouge as women. Vanity was gender-neutral, and so was the poisoning.

And yet, no public regulation existed to restrict or ban mercury in cosmetics. The pursuit of beauty, status, and visibility trumped emerging medical warnings. The danger was known but ignored,an echo we still hear today.

This Roman chapter reveals a core truth: when beauty is tied to status, health becomes collateral damage. It's a lesson the modern world continues to relearn, too often at the cost of our bodies.

Romans were obsessed with appearances. Pale skin signified status, leisure, and affluence. And so, mercury-based creams became the go-to for lightening the face. The side effects included neurological damage, chronic fatigue, reproductive disorders, and hallucinations. All masked under the rouge and powder. Even the men of Rome indulged in these deadly potions. Beauty was gendered, but poison was equal-opportunity (Dunn, 1994).

Renaissance & Victorian Eras: Arsenic, Belladonna, and Broken Bodies

The Renaissance period ushered in a renewed fascination with art, symmetry, and the human form. But this so-called enlightenment also brought with it dangerous beauty practices disguised as refinement. Among the elite, the ideal woman was fair-skinned, wide-eyed, and porcelain-pale-so pale, in fact, that it suggested illness, fragility, and a life untouched by labor or sun.

To achieve this aesthetic, women turned to some of the most toxic substances available.

Belladonna, also known as "deadly nightshade," was used as an eye drop to dilate the pupils and give the wearer a romantic, doe-eyed appearance. The name itself, "beautiful woman" in Italian, speaks to its cosmetic value. But its effects were far from harmless. Prolonged use led to blurred vision, light sensitivity, and in many cases, permanent eye damage or blindness. Women chose visual deterioration in exchange for visual appeal.

At the same time, arsenic became a go-to solution for pale, luminous skin. Arsenic wafers and tonics were sold as ingestible complexion enhancers. These products promised to erase blemishes, lighten skin, and give the user a delicate, almost ethereal glow. What they actually did was damage internal organs, cause nausea and vomiting, thin the hair, and eventually lead to organ failure. Some formulas included just enough arsenic to produce short-term effects, keeping customers dependent without killing them too quickly. These weren't just vanity tools; they were slow poisons with mass appeal.

Moving into the Victorian era, the obsession with whiteness and delicacy deepened. The industrial revolution brought new chemicals and mass production, which meant that toxic beauty was no longer reserved for the wealthy. Middle-class women now had access to a growing array of powders, creams, and complexion pills laced with ammonia, chalk, lead, and mercury.

"Complexion wafers", paper-thin tablets containing arsenic and other whiteners were marketed in women's magazines as essential tools for maintaining a ladylike appearance. These wafers, when combined with tight corsetry and layers of restrictive clothing, created a perfect storm of systemic stress. Corsets compressed internal organs, limited oxygen, and caused chronic fainting.

Women's bodies became the canvas for a cruel cultural ideal: the more frail and breakable she appeared, the more she fit the mold.

The Victorian ideal of beauty was paradoxical: it celebrated the look of health through the visible signs of illness. A fevered blush, pale lips, thin waists, and fainting spells were not red flags-they were goals. Women powdered their faces with lead, knowing it made their skin dry and pale. They inhaled ammonia to stay awake and alert despite chronic fatigue. They traded strength for style, agency for aesthetics.

This era left behind more than paintings and poetry. It left a legacy of generational beauty trauma; a normalization of self-harm in the name of social acceptance. And although the powders may have changed, the pressure to contort ourselves into idealized versions of beauty remains.

When we look back at the arsenic and belladonna era, we're tempted to scoff, to say, "How could they not have known?" But the truth is, many *did* know. They were simply taught to ignore their instincts. Just as many of us still are today.

20th Century: Glow-in-the-Dark Girls and Mascara Blindness

The turn of the 20th century brought with it rapid technological advancement and industrial optimism. Science and innovation promised to solve all problems-even aging. And nowhere was this promise more dangerously misapplied than in the world of cosmetics.

By the early 1900s, radium-a radioactive element discovered in the late 1800s-was seen as a miracle cure. Its faint, ghostly glow and novelty status made it appealing to the public, and beauty companies quickly capitalized. Radium was marketed as rejuvenating, detoxifying, and life-giving. Face creams, powders, and tonics laced with radium hit store shelves with glamorous packaging and bold claims.

These products were not reserved for elites. Everyday women, drawn by the allure of modern beauty science, began applying radium-laced creams to their skin. It was believed to smooth wrinkles, enhance the complexion, and restore vitality. In reality, it was a death sentence. Radiation breaks down cellular structures, damages DNA, and causes deep internal damage long before external symptoms appear.

The most infamous victims were the "Radium Girls"-young factory workers hired to paint glowing numbers on watch dials using luminescent paint made with radium. They were instructed to "lip-point" their brushes, shaping the tips with their tongues. Day after day, they ingested radioactive particles. Their teeth fell out. Their bones crumbled. Their jaws deteriorated. Many died slow, painful deaths, all while the companies denied any link to their products (Clark, 1997).

These tragedies eventually led to landmark labor lawsuits and increased public scrutiny, but the cosmetic industry escaped most of the blame. Radium remained in certain beauty products well into the 1930s.

Then came Lash Lure.

In 1933, a new mascara product entered the market, promising lush, dramatic lashes. Lash Lure contained p-phenylenediamine, a coal tar-derived dye known to cause severe allergic reactions. Women who used it experienced swelling, blistering, permanent eye damage, and even death. One woman, Mabel Green, died after using the product for a wedding. The resulting outrage was one of the few moments in U.S. history where cosmetic regulation was seriously debated.

Despite the tragic outcomes, the product was not immediately pulled from shelves. There was no federal law requiring safety testing before cosmetics hit the market. In fact, it took years of public pressure before even basic legislation-the 1938 Federal Food, Drug, and Cosmetic Act-was passed. And even then, the new law offered minimal oversight for cosmetics compared to food and drugs.

The stories of the Radium Girls and the victims of Lash Lure reveal the same pattern: untested innovation, corporate denial, regulatory apathy, and preventable harm. These women were collateral damage in a system that valued profit over protection.

These chapters of cosmetic history are not distant. They're foundational. And unless we remember them, we risk repeating them. The products may look cleaner today, but the lack of oversight remains disturbingly familiar.

Today: Pretty Lies in Plastic Bottles

Fast forward to today, and it might seem like we should know better. The lessons of radium and lead should have taught us something. But we are still applying known endocrine disruptors, carcinogens, and allergens every single day. The difference now is that the poison is wrapped in prettier packaging, and it's endorsed by celebrities.

From phthalates to parabens, formaldehyde to "fragrance," the industry hides toxins behind long words and tiny print. The term "fragrance" alone can include hundreds of undisclosed chemicals, many of them hormone disruptors (EWG, 2021). And worse, the FDA allows it. The U.S. cosmetic industry is largely self-regulated. Companies are not required to prove safety before going to market. And they do not.

Beauty has never truly been about health. It has been about control. About profit. About keeping women-and increasingly men-on the treadmill of not quite enough. A billion-dollar industry profits off insecurity, then sells chemical solutions.

The truth they will not sell you is this: real beauty does not cost your health. Real radiance starts from within. It begins with a nourished body, balanced hormones, clean skin, and truth.

This truth has been buried, but we are digging it up. And in the next chapter, we'll uncover one of the most insidious tools the industry ever created: the invention of flaws.

CHAPTER 2:

The Invention of Flaws

There was a time when freckles were kissed by the sun, when wrinkles were seen as earned wisdom, and when aging was not something to fight, but something to embrace. That time is gone. Today, most women, and increasingly men, are taught to spot their first flaw before they're even old enough to vote. The wrinkle, the pore, the line, the bump, the "imperfection."

But where did this obsession come from? Why do we look at our bodies and see a list of problems to solve?

The short answer: we were taught to. The long answer: we were sold to.

Selling Insecurity: A Business Model

In the early 20th century, advertising shifted dramatically. Rather than selling products based on utility, companies began to sell desire, and more powerfully, fear. The emerging beauty industry realized that in order to grow, it couldn't just sell lipstick. It had to sell the need for lipstick. That meant creating problems where there weren't any. Suddenly, pores became a flaw. Gray hair was unacceptable. Natural skin texture became something to "treat."

Edward Bernays, the so-called "father of public relations," was instrumental in this shift. In the 1920s, he helped transform cigarettes into a symbol of female independence. He also consulted for cosmetic companies, helping to craft messaging that tied products to identity, status, and worth (Tye, 1998). The implication was clear:

beauty was no longer optional. It was currency, and it came with a cost.

This shift wasn't subtle. It was aggressive, strategic, and deeply effective. By the 1950s, the average American woman owned multiple cosmetic products and felt pressured to maintain a polished appearance even at home. Ads in women's magazines promoted creams to eliminate "crow's feet," tonics to reduce "unsightly blemishes," and powders to "refine" the skin. These ads didn't merely present options, they planted seeds of inadequacy. They turned natural features into liabilities and aging into a disease to be treated.

Beauty became a system of consumption and conformity, reinforced through imagery, repetition, and peer pressure. If you wanted to be desirable, you had to participate. If you opted out, you risked social invisibility.

From Observation to Obsession

This wasn't just marketing. It became cultural programming. Generations of girls grew up watching their mothers apologize for their faces, conceal their fatigue, and fear aging. "I look tired," became a moral failing. "I need to fix my face," became normal. Cosmetics, originally used as adornment, were now reframed as maintenance. Flaws were to be fought, not accepted.

The obsession with flaws mutated over time. In the 1980s, the beauty industry discovered a goldmine in anti-aging. Products that promised to "reverse time" hit the shelves, capitalizing on the growing fear of looking older. Wrinkles were pathologized. Sagging skin was shameful. Age spots were targeted like a public health threat. Skincare transformed into a war zone, with "miracle" creams and "dermatologist-approved" solutions acting as the weapons.

By the 2000s, the rise of high-definition television and social media filters created a new epidemic: hyper-visibility. Skin was now expected to look like porcelain under a microscope. Pores had to disappear. Lines were a threat. Any deviation from the airbrushed ideal was now considered a flaw. The result was a collective dissociation from reality. Real skin, with texture and variation, became something to hide.

The worst part? None of it was rooted in health. In fact, many of the products sold to address these so-called flaws contained toxins, allergens, and hormone disruptors. What was presented as care was actually sabotage.

The Rise of "Fix Culture"

The psychological toll of beauty obsession cannot be overstated. Beneath the surface rituals and aesthetic upgrades lies a much deeper emotional cost. As beauty has become more synonymous with self-worth, the pressure to perfect has become internalized to the point of pathology.

Rates of body dysmorphia, anxiety, and depression have climbed alongside the rise in cosmetic procedures and social media filters. Constant comparison, both in private mirrors and public feeds, has normalized chronic dissatisfaction with one's appearance. Studies show that individuals, especially women, who frequently engage with beauty-related content are more likely to experience low self-esteem, heightened anxiety, and disordered eating patterns.

Social media platforms, which were originally meant to connect us, have amplified this issue. Algorithms reward curated perfection and filtered illusions, making the average person's unedited face feel inadequate. The result is a feedback loop of self-surveillance, where beauty becomes an ongoing project and our mental health becomes collateral damage.

This culture of constant fixing rewires the brain. Neuroplasticity means that repeated thoughts and behaviors form well-worn pathways. The more we focus on our "flaws," the deeper those grooves become, until even moments of quiet are filled with the static of self-criticism. This chronic stress impacts the nervous system, affects sleep, raises cortisol, and contributes to inflammation, not just emotionally, but physically.

The mental health crisis tethered to beauty culture isn't simply about wanting to look good. It's about a culture that teaches us that *not looking good* is a problem so profound, it must be solved through consumption. And because perfection is always just out of reach, the chase never ends.

Fix culture is not just exhausting. It is depleting. It narrows our focus until we forget what else we could be using our minds, our energy, and our lives for.

From Botox to filters to thousand-dollar skincare routines, the modern face is now a battleground. We're no longer aging, we're "fighting" age. We're not applying makeup, we're "correcting" features. What was once an adornment has become armor. And underneath it, many women are left feeling disconnected from their real faces, their real beauty, and their real bodies.

This constant fixing doesn't end at the surface. It rewires the nervous system. It heightens cortisol. It drives anxiety, body dysmorphia, and disordered habits. The message is clear: you are not enough until you buy your way there.

The beauty industry is not just profiting off your desire to look good. It is profiting off your deepest fears, fear of rejection, of invisibility, of aging, of not being loved. And it packages those fears into products with expiration dates, ensuring that you always need more.

And that message, repeated long enough, becomes internalized. It becomes the new normal. It becomes a silent contract we sign without realizing, agreeing to perform a version of ourselves that is more palatable, more polished, more profitable.

But it doesn't have to be.

There is another way. One rooted in truth, in health, and in rebellion against the commodification of your face. In the next chapter, we'll examine how regulation, or the lack of it, has allowed harmful products to flood the market. We'll look at the real policies and the hidden loopholes that keep toxic ingredients on store shelves and in our homes.

CHAPTER 3:

Beautifully Unregulated

We like to think someone's watching out for us. That the lotions we slather on our skin, the lipsticks we press to our mouths, and the serums we dab near our eyes are safe because they're *allowed* on the shelf. There must be testing, oversight, some kind of protective system in place... right?

The uncomfortable truth is this: in the United States, the cosmetics industry is one of the least regulated industries in the consumer space. And for decades, it has stayed that way, not by accident, but by careful design. Loopholes, lobbying, and a lack of public awareness have created a regulatory environment that favors corporations, not consumers.

A Toothless Guardian: The FDA's Limited Role

The Food and Drug Administration (FDA), the federal agency responsible for protecting public health, does not pre-approve cosmetics before they go to market. Unlike pharmaceuticals or even certain food additives, cosmetic products are not required to undergo any safety testing prior to being sold to the public. The FDA has no authority to demand recalls and cannot mandate reformulations unless serious harm has been demonstrated.

Instead, manufacturers are expected to self-regulate. They choose their own safety standards, perform their own testing, and determine what information to share with consumers. If that sounds like a conflict of interest, it is because it is. There is no independent verification, no pre-market approval, and minimal post-market accountability.

To make matters worse, only 11 cosmetic ingredients are currently banned or restricted by law in the United States. In contrast, the European Union has banned or restricted over 1,300 ingredients. This vast difference highlights just how lenient the American system is when it comes to chemical safety in personal care.

One of the most egregious loopholes is the use of the term "fragrance." Companies are not legally required to disclose the individual ingredients in a product's fragrance formula. This single word can conceal hundreds of different chemicals, including known allergens, hormone disruptors, and even carcinogens (EWG, 2021).

The Power of "Fragrance" and Trade Secrets

The word "fragrance" may seem innocent-just a pleasant smell, a signature scent, or a little luxury added to a product. But behind that single word lies one of the largest loopholes in the modern cosmetic industry.

Legally, "fragrance" is considered a trade secret, meaning manufacturers are not required to disclose the actual chemical composition of any ingredient labeled as such. This protection was originally intended to safeguard proprietary perfume blends from being copied by competitors. However, in practice, it has allowed companies to hide hundreds of potentially toxic chemicals from consumers without consequence.

What does this mean in reality? It means that you could be using a face cream, shampoo, deodorant, or baby product containing dozens of undisclosed substances, some of which may be allergens, irritants, hormone disruptors, or even carcinogens, and you would have no way of knowing.

One of the most commonly concealed families of chemicals under "fragrance" are phthalates. These are plasticizers used to help scents last longer on the skin or in the air. Phthalates have been linked to serious health issues including endocrine disruption, reduced sperm quality, impaired fetal development, and increased risk of asthma and allergic disease in children. And yet, they are rarely listed on any product label because they are embedded within the legally protected "fragrance" mixture.

This kind of ingredient masking is not rare, it is standard. It applies to products marketed to all demographics, including those labeled as "natural," "clean," or "eco-conscious."

To complicate matters further, many products labeled as "unscented" still contain fragrance chemicals. These are known as masking agents, and they are added not to provide a scent, but to neutralize other smells within the formulation. Again, these are hidden under the same blanket term: "fragrance."

What makes this issue particularly insidious is how difficult it is for consumers to make informed choices. Even highly motivated, ingredient-savvy shoppers cannot decode what's behind "fragrance." There is no access to a full list of what's inside, no regulatory requirement to test these chemicals for safety in combination, and no warning labels indicating potential health effects.

In effect, the word "fragrance" functions as a legal blindfold. It allows brands to retain a facade of sophistication and scent while avoiding transparency. Meanwhile, the burden of risk falls entirely on the consumer. If a product causes irritation, disrupts hormones, or contributes to long-term disease, the manufacturer is rarely held accountable. There are no mandated disclosures, no proactive warnings, and no meaningful regulation forcing companies to reformulate.

Until legislation changes, "fragrance" will remain one of the most effective tools companies use to bypass scrutiny. It is a loophole that smells sweet but masks a bitter truth.

Self-Policing in a Billion-Dollar Industry

The primary body that oversees cosmetic ingredient safety in the United States is the Cosmetic Ingredient Review (CIR) panel. On paper, this might sound like a legitimate scientific watchdog. In reality, the CIR is funded and operated by the Personal Care Products Council-a powerful industry trade association representing some of the biggest names in beauty and personal care. This inherent conflict of interest severely undermines the credibility and independence of the panel's reviews.

While the CIR does publish safety assessments and recommends ingredient restrictions or usage guidelines, it has no legal authority. Compliance with its findings is entirely voluntary. Companies can, and often do ignore its recommendations without fear of enforcement, penalty, or even public disclosure. This setup allows companies to present an image of oversight while continuing to use potentially harmful ingredients in their formulations.

This voluntary, industry-led model is what makes the cosmetic sector so vulnerable to abuses of power. Unlike pharmaceuticals, which must pass rigorous clinical trials, cosmetics are considered low-risk products and are therefore exempt from many of the basic safety protocols required in other health-related industries. Yet the irony is clear: these so-called "low-risk" products are applied daily, often multiple times a day, directly to the body's largest organ: our skin. And many contain ingredients that are known endocrine disruptors, allergens, or sensitizers.

When a product causes harm, be it a rash, hormonal imbalance, hair loss, or worse, the burden of proof is placed on the consumer. The FDA receives thousands of complaints each year about cosmetic-related injuries or illnesses, but it lacks both the staff and the statutory power to investigate most of them meaningfully. Unless an issue garners significant media attention or results in a lawsuit, the agency has no obligation to act. In the rare instances when it does, action tends to be slow, limited, and reactive rather than preventative.

What this means is that the system depends on consumer harm and subsequent public outrage to prompt any corrective measures. It is not a safety-first model. It is a crisis-response model, one that inherently favors corporate interests over public well-being. In a billion-dollar industry driven by marketing, image, and speed to shelf, this lack of mandatory accountability is not just a regulatory flaw, it is a systemic failure.

The result? A market flooded with products that prioritize profit over safety, where innovation is measured by how quickly a trend can be monetized, not by how well a product supports health. Until this model changes, consumers are left to navigate a treacherous landscape of self-policing corporations and silent regulators, armed with little more than their instincts, a smartphone app, and the hope that the label tells the truth.

The Politics of Beauty and Influence

Behind this lax regulatory landscape lies a complex and well-funded network of political influence. Major cosmetic and personal care corporations spend millions of dollars each year lobbying members of Congress, funding trade associations, and shaping regulatory outcomes in their favor. These efforts are not just reactive-they are proactive, designed to block consumer protections before they even gain momentum.

One of the clearest examples of this influence is the repeated stalling and failure of the Safe Cosmetics and Personal Care Products Act. First introduced in 2010, and reintroduced multiple times in the years that followed, this bill aimed to give the FDA more power to review ingredients, mandate recalls, and enforce safety standards. However, it never made it past committee. Lobbying from industry giants like Procter & Gamble, Johnson & Johnson, and Estée Lauder ensured that momentum for the bill fizzled out, time and again.

These companies argue that stricter regulations would hinder innovation or increase costs for consumers, but such claims often obscure the true motive: protecting profit. The cosmetic industry is projected to exceed $600 billion globally by 2030. In this high-stakes market, any regulation that increases transparency or demands ingredient safety threatens not just product lines-but entire brand identities built on aspirational marketing.

Real-life consequences of this influence have surfaced repeatedly. Consider the Johnson & Johnson talcum powder scandal. For decades, the company marketed its baby powder as pure and gentle, while internal documents later revealed that executives were aware of asbestos contamination risks as early as the 1970s. It was not until thousands of lawsuits and a 2018 investigative report by Reuters that public awareness exploded. In 2020, Johnson & Johnson pulled talc-based baby powder from U.S. shelves-not because of FDA enforcement, but due to mounting legal and consumer pressure. The product is still sold in other countries.

This case underscores the power of political protection. Despite long-standing safety concerns and legal battles, the product remained on the market, and the company faced minimal regulatory consequences. Only mass litigation and media exposure created enough momentum for change.

This is not an isolated case. From hair straighteners linked to hormone disruption to skin lightening creams containing mercury, the cosmetic industry's track record is riddled with examples where corporate influence delayed or denied accountability. These products disproportionately impact vulnerable populations, including Black and brown communities, further illustrating how regulatory inaction can reinforce systemic inequities.

There is money to be made in opacity. Transparency invites scrutiny, and scrutiny leads to accountability. For an industry built on aspirational marketing, brand loyalty, and carefully curated illusions, exposure is not just inconvenient-it is dangerous.

Until legislation is driven by independent science rather than corporate interests, consumers will continue to pay the price-not just at the register, but in long-term health consequences that could have been prevented.

Behind this lax regulatory landscape lies a complex web of political influence. Major cosmetic companies spend millions of dollars each year on lobbying efforts to protect their interests and prevent stricter regulations.

Attempts to pass comprehensive safety legislation, such as the Safe Cosmetics and Personal Care Products Act, have repeatedly failed to gain traction in Congress. Industry lobbyists argue that new regulations would stifle innovation and burden small businesses, but in reality, these objections protect profit margins at the expense of public health.

There is money to be made in opacity. Transparency invites scrutiny, and scrutiny leads to accountability. For an industry built on aspirational marketing and brand loyalty, exposure is a threat.

Regulatory Theater and Greenwashing

In recent years, as public awareness around toxic ingredients has grown, beauty companies have been forced to adapt. Consumers are reading labels more carefully, asking questions about what they put on their skin, and seeking out safer options. But rather than changing harmful formulations, many brands have leaned into a marketing strategy that offers the appearance of change without the substance. This is the heart of regulatory theater and greenwashing.

Greenwashing refers to the practice of making products appear more environmentally friendly or health-conscious than they actually are. In the cosmetics world, it often shows up as packaging that features leaves, water droplets, and earthy tones. Products are marketed using buzzwords like "natural," "clean," "non-toxic," "pure," or "eco," even when their ingredient lists contain synthetic preservatives, harsh surfactants, or known irritants. These terms are largely unregulated and have no standardized definitions under U.S. law. As a result, companies are free to use them however they choose.

For example, a moisturizer labeled as "natural" might still contain petrochemicals, artificial dyes, and preservatives like phenoxyethanol. A product labeled "hypoallergenic" can legally contain common allergens and irritants. "Non-toxic" sounds reassuring but has no legally binding meaning in this context. And "dermatologist-tested" simply means that a dermatologist looked at or used the product; it does not mean the product is free from harmful ingredients or that it passed rigorous safety trials.

This form of branding is not accidental. It is part of a broader public relations effort designed to meet consumer demand for safety without compromising the industry's profit-driven formulas. Regulatory theater gives consumers the illusion of oversight while allowing manufacturers to continue business as usual.

A real-life example of greenwashing can be found in products marketed as "paraben-free" or "sulfate-free." While removing parabens or sulfates might sound like progress, many brands simply replace these ingredients with other synthetic chemicals that have not been thoroughly tested for long-term safety. For instance, methylisothiazolinone is a common preservative used in place of parabens, yet it has been associated with skin irritation and allergic reactions. But because it is not a "paraben," it often flies under the radar.

Even certification labels can be misleading. Some brands create their own in-house certification icons that resemble third-party approvals, such as leaves or badges that say "green certified" or "clean formula." These labels may not correspond to any recognized safety standards and are used primarily to create a sense of trust.

The result is a consumer landscape where even well-meaning individuals can be easily misled. Shoppers who want to make better choices are frequently undermined by confusing language, clever packaging, and the absence of meaningful regulation. Without legal accountability, the responsibility for deciphering truth from marketing falls entirely on the public.

True change requires more than label makeovers. It demands transparency, standardized definitions, mandatory safety testing, and third-party verification. Until these are in place, greenwashing will continue to flourish, and consumers will remain vulnerable to the very risks they are trying to avoid.

This form of regulatory theater is designed to soothe concerns without making meaningful changes. It gives the illusion of safety while allowing harmful ingredients to remain.

Why the Burden Falls on You

In the absence of strong oversight, the responsibility for safety has shifted to the consumer. Shoppers are expected to become amateur chemists-reading labels, researching compounds, and evaluating risks on their own. This is not only unrealistic, but deeply unfair.

Most people do not have the time, training, or resources to vet every ingredient in every product they use. And even those who try are often thwarted by vague terminology, proprietary formulas, and hidden chemicals.

In a just system, safety would be the default, not a luxury. Ingredient transparency would be standard. Products would be tested for long-term health impacts, not just short-term results. Companies would be held accountable for harm.

But we do not live in that system. We live in one where marketing often carries more weight than medicine, and where the illusion of regulation masks a troubling reality.

In the next chapter, we'll explore what these ingredients are actually doing inside your body. We'll take a closer look at endocrine disruptors, carcinogens, and allergens found in everyday products, and uncover how they're impacting our hormones, fertility, and long-term health.

CHAPTER 4:

Hormones Hijacked

Every day, we interact with beauty products that promise to nourish, revitalize, and beautify. But what they are really doing is far more insidious. Hidden inside the average skincare routine are compounds that quietly interfere with the body's most delicate and essential signaling system: the endocrine system.

The endocrine system does not just regulate reproductive health. It affects nearly every system in the body. Hormones influence your mood, metabolism, energy levels, cognitive function, fertility, immunity, and how your body responds to stress and aging. And every day, that intricate hormonal dance is being disrupted by chemicals in products that most people believe are safe.

The Role of the Endocrine System

The endocrine system is composed of glands such as the thyroid, pituitary, adrenal glands, ovaries, and testes, which secrete hormones that act like chemical messengers. These hormones are sent through the bloodstream to tissues and organs, telling them what to do and when to do it. The balance of these hormones is finely tuned and highly sensitive to disruption.

Even minor hormonal imbalances can lead to fatigue, weight gain, sleep disturbances, menstrual irregularities, mood swings, low libido, infertility, immune dysfunction, and increased risk for chronic illness. When this system is hijacked by external synthetic chemicals, the body is forced to compensate, adapt, or break down entirely.

Endocrine-disrupting chemicals (EDCs) can mimic, block, or alter these hormonal messages. They may look similar to natural hormones like estrogen or testosterone, tricking the body into responding to them, or they may prevent actual hormones from binding to their receptors. What makes EDCs especially harmful is that their effects are often non-linear: even low doses can cause significant biological changes, especially with chronic exposure over time (Vandenberg et al., 2012).

The Big Offenders

Let's break down some of the most common and dangerous EDCs found in cosmetics and personal care products:

- Phthalates: Often found in fragrance blends, hair sprays, and nail polishes. Linked to decreased testosterone levels, reduced sperm quality, altered genital development in male infants, and increased risk of asthma and allergies in children.

- Parabens: Used as preservatives in lotions, shampoos, and makeup. Known to mimic estrogen and have been detected in breast tumor tissue (Darbre et al., 2004). They are associated with early puberty and disrupted menstrual cycles.

- Oxybenzone: A chemical commonly used in sunscreens. It acts as a hormone disruptor and allergen. Oxybenzone has been shown to interfere with estrogen, androgen, and thyroid hormone signaling, especially concerning for pregnant women and developing fetuses (Krause et al., 2012).

- Triclosan: Previously common in antibacterial soaps and toothpaste. Shown to interfere with thyroid hormone metabolism and potentially impair immune function.

- Formaldehyde and formaldehyde-releasing preservatives: Found in some hair straightening products and nail treatments. These chemicals are known carcinogens and skin sensitizers.

These chemicals do not remain on the skin's surface. Many of them are lipophilic, which means they are fat-soluble and can dissolve into the fatty tissues of the body. This property allows them to accumulate in areas such as the breasts, reproductive organs, liver, and brain, areas that are highly sensitive to hormonal signaling. Once stored in adipose tissue, these chemicals can slowly leach into the bloodstream over time, extending their influence well beyond the moment of application.

Additionally, their molecular structure is often small and synthetic enough to penetrate the skin barrier with ease. Once inside the body, they enter the circulatory system, where they are distributed to tissues and organs. From there, they may interact directly with hormone receptors or compete with natural hormones, causing confusion at the cellular level. Some of these compounds have been shown in laboratory and epidemiological studies to cross the blood-brain barrier, a highly selective membrane designed to protect the brain from toxins. Their presence in the central nervous system raises concern about long-term effects on cognition, mood regulation, and neurological development.

Even more concerning is emerging research that suggests certain endocrine-disrupting chemicals may influence epigenetic activity. This means they could alter how genes are expressed without changing the DNA sequence itself, potentially impacting not only the exposed individual but also future generations. These intergenerational effects make the long-term risks of daily cosmetic exposure especially urgent to address.

The Problem with "Safe Doses"

A common industry defense is that these ingredients appear in products at "safe levels." But this argument fails for three reasons:

1. Bioaccumulation: The body may be exposed to small doses from individual products, but when those products are used daily and across multiple categories—shampoo, lotion, makeup, deodorant—the exposure adds up. These chemicals accumulate over time and may not be efficiently cleared by the liver or kidneys.

2. Chemical cocktails: Real life does not mimic lab studies. People are not exposed to isolated substances in controlled environments. Instead, we are bombarded with complex mixtures of chemicals from hundreds of products. The synergistic or combined effects of multiple EDCs interacting

in the body are largely unknown and rarely studied.

3. Sensitive populations: Fetuses, infants, children, and those with existing hormonal conditions are more vulnerable to the effects of EDCs. What may be considered "safe" for a healthy adult male might be deeply disruptive to a developing fetus or someone with a thyroid condition.

The reality is that most of the safety data used to justify continued use of these chemicals is severely lacking in scope, depth, and modern relevance. Much of this data stems from studies conducted decades ago, using methodologies that do not reflect how people actually use personal care products today. These studies often focus on isolated compounds tested in laboratory conditions, examining short-term exposure in adult animals or cell cultures. They rarely consider the cumulative, daily exposure most individuals experience through the use of multiple products across a variety of categories, from shampoo to deodorant to cosmetics. Nor do they account for vulnerable populations such as infants, pregnant women, or individuals with chronic health conditions.

Even more troubling is that very few of these studies investigate the effects of chemical mixtures, despite the fact that consumers are exposed to dozens or even hundreds of synthetic ingredients every day. This chemical cocktail effect is poorly understood, but early research suggests that these interactions may amplify the toxic effects of individual ingredients. Moreover, most safety assessments completely ignore the possibility of transgenerational harm. Emerging studies in the field of epigenetics indicate that exposure to endocrine-disrupting chemicals can alter gene expression in ways that may affect not just the individual, but their children and grandchildren as well.

In other words, the existing data used to defend these chemicals often fails to reflect real-world conditions, does not account for chronic or compounding exposure, and is not designed to identify long-term, low-dose effects. Without updated, rigorous, and independent research that includes modern usage patterns and multi-generational impacts, the claim of "safe levels" remains scientifically unsubstantiated and ethically irresponsible.

Real Consequences, Real People

The consequences of chronic exposure to endocrine-disrupting chemicals are no longer abstract. They are manifesting in real people, across generations, in ways that are reshaping public health as we know it.

- Early puberty: Today, many girls are entering puberty as early as age 8. This shift is not merely a curiosity, it is a biological alarm bell. Early onset of puberty has been linked to a higher risk of breast cancer, emotional distress, and lifelong hormonal instability. EDCs that mimic estrogen are primary suspects, and they are showing up in urine samples of young children.

- Infertility: The World Health Organization now recognizes infertility as a global health issue. Male fertility has declined sharply, with studies showing sperm counts dropping by more than half since the 1970s (Levine et al., 2017). Many scientists believe that exposure to environmental toxins, especially phthalates and BPA, plays a significant role. In women, rising cases of PCOS, unexplained infertility, and miscarriage are increasingly tied to chronic low-dose exposure to EDCs.

- Endocrine-related diseases: Endometriosis, thyroid disorders, fibroids, breast and testicular cancers, these conditions are on the rise, and while they may have multiple causes, EDCs are consistently implicated as contributing or exacerbating factors. These are not niche concerns. They are widespread and growing. According to the Endocrine Society, there is strong evidence linking EDC exposure to hormonal cancers, metabolic diseases, and reproductive harm.

- Neurodevelopmental disorders: Perhaps most sobering is the growing body of research linking prenatal exposure to EDCs with developmental and cognitive impairments. Chemicals like BPA and phthalates are found in nearly every person tested, including pregnant women. These compounds can pass through the placenta and influence fetal brain development. Children exposed in utero may face increased risk of ADHD, anxiety, autism spectrum disorder, and reduced IQ.

- Intergenerational effects: These health impacts are not always limited to the exposed individual. Animal studies and early human research suggest that the effects of EDCs can echo across generations. This means that a pregnant woman's exposure today could influence her grandchildren's hormonal, neurological, or reproductive health through epigenetic changes.

These are not isolated incidents or rare outcomes. They are patterns, and they are worsening. Yet most people remain unaware that the lotion they apply, the shampoo they use, or the lipstick they wear could be contributing to a spectrum of lifelong, systemic health challenges. The disconnect between everyday routines and chronic disease is not just tragic, it is engineered through silence, marketing, and a failure of public health messaging.

We are not just talking about inconvenience. We are talking about a slow erosion of biological resilience. These chemicals chip away at the body's ability to regulate itself, reproduce healthfully, and protect future generations. That is the true cost of beauty when its definition is dictated by unregulated, profit-driven industries.

It Is Not Just a "Women's Issue"

Hormonal disruption affects everyone. While much of the marketing and media focus is placed on women and beauty, EDCs do not discriminate. Men are experiencing declines in testosterone, lower sperm motility, erectile dysfunction, and increased incidence of testicular cancer. Children are born already carrying measurable levels of synthetic chemicals passed through the placenta or breast milk.

And yet, most of the public discourse around EDCs remains centered on women's products and framed in beauty terms. This minimizes the issue and misses the broader, more urgent point: this is not about vanity. It is about the health of entire populations.

Rebuilding Hormonal Safety

So where do we begin?

The first step is not to panic. It is *awareness*. Becoming informed about the risks is the beginning of empowerment. The next step is simplification. Removing unnecessary products from your routine is not a sacrifice, it is a liberation.

Start with a few high-impact changes:

- Avoid anything with "fragrance" or "parfum" on the label.

- Switch to mineral-based sunscreens using zinc oxide or titanium dioxide.

- Replace conventional lotions with tallow-based or single-ingredient oils.

- Use glass or stainless steel containers to reduce plastic leaching.

- Prioritize brands with third-party safety certifications like EWG Verified or Made Safe.

Ultimately, choose ancestral, bio-compatible ingredients. Your skin does not need complexity, it needs nourishment. What you put on your skin should support, not sabotage, the internal systems your body relies on to function.

Your skin is not just a canvas for beauty. It is an organ. It is porous. It communicates with your brain, your hormones, and your immune system. Treating it with respect is not a luxury. It is foundational health.

Helpful tip: don't put something on your skin that you wouldn't eat. It's that connected.

In the next chapter, we will explore what happens when these internal hormonal disruptions start to manifest externally. Acne, eczema, rashes, and inflammation are not just cosmetic issues. They are signals. We will connect the dots between product choices, internal imbalance, and the visible signs that something deeper is out of sync.

CHAPTER 5:

Skin Deep Symptoms

When we think of skincare, we often envision radiance, glow, and clarity. Marketing images show smooth, glowing complexions and the promise of transformation. But more and more people, especially women, are waking up to skin that feels inflamed, irritated, and reactive. Despite spending hundreds or even thousands of dollars on skincare products, the results are often worse, not better. Skin doesn't get calmer. It gets angrier.

The irony is stark. Many of the very products that promise healing and rejuvenation are actually causing the issues they claim to fix. This is not just marketing misdirection. It is a public health issue.

When the Skin Speaks

The skin is the body's largest organ. It is not just a passive surface. It serves as a physical barrier, an immune responder, a detox pathway, and a vital part of the body's communication system. It reacts to both internal imbalances and external insults. When it breaks out, flakes, burns, or reacts, it is trying to tell us something. The problem is that most of us have been taught to silence those signals with concealer, acid peels, and steroid creams.

Let's explore some of the most common skin symptoms linked to modern cosmetic use and what they might actually be revealing:

Acne and Cystic Breakouts

Adult acne is on the rise, especially among women over the age of 25. This is no longer considered just a teenage issue. A growing body of evidence links persistent breakouts to hormonal imbalances, many of which are driven by endocrine-disrupting chemicals in cosmetics. Parabens, phthalates, and synthetic fragrances can mimic hormones and disrupt the delicate balance of estrogen, testosterone, and progesterone.

In addition, many mainstream products are loaded with pore-clogging agents like silicones, waxes, and petroleum derivatives. Over-cleansing, exfoliating, and applying too many actives can strip the skin's protective barrier, leading to inflammation, bacterial overgrowth, and more acne. Dermatological interventions often focus on symptom suppression, antibiotics, benzoyl peroxide, or retinoids, without addressing the root causes or the product exposures that may be contributing to the problem.

Rashes, Eczema, and Dermatitis

Skin rashes are more than surface irritation. They are signs of deeper immune dysregulation. Contact dermatitis, for instance, is one of the fastest-growing diagnoses in dermatology, and many cases are traced back to ingredients found in everyday personal care products.

Common culprits include:

- Fragrance chemicals, which can trigger allergic reactions and are often labeled vaguely as "parfum" or "natural scent."

- Methylisothiazolinone, a widely used preservative that has been flagged by the American Contact Dermatitis Society as a top allergen.

- Formaldehyde-releasing compounds, used to extend shelf life, which can cause chronic irritation and sensitization over time.

These skin issues are often managed with topical steroids, which may reduce inflammation temporarily but do not remove the underlying trigger. Prolonged steroid use can further weaken the skin barrier and contribute to thinning, discoloration, and increased susceptibility to flare-ups.

Autoimmune Skin Disorders

Conditions like psoriasis, rosacea, and lupus-related rashes are complex and multifactorial, but research increasingly shows that environmental toxins, including those in personal care products, can exacerbate these autoimmune conditions. In people whose immune systems are already dysregulated, adding a daily dose of synthetic irritants and hormone disruptors may heighten systemic inflammation and trigger more frequent or intense flare-ups.

Premature Aging

Ironically, many so-called anti-aging products accelerate the very aging process they promise to reverse. Harsh exfoliants, alcohol-based toners, synthetic retinoids, and alpha hydroxy acids can degrade the skin barrier over time, leaving it dry, thin, and more prone to sun damage.

This chronic irritation leads to:

- Increased transepidermal water loss (TEWL)

- Collagen breakdown

- Hyperpigmentation and uneven tone

- Heightened sensitivity to ultraviolet (UV) radiation

Rather than restoring youthfulness, these products can initiate a cycle of damage and dependency, where the skin becomes increasingly fragile and reliant on products to compensate for its lost resilience.

The Gut-Skin Connection

The relationship between gut health and skin health is not merely a theory; it is a complex, well-documented physiological connection supported by both ancient holistic practices and modern biomedical science. The gut and the skin are two of the body's primary detoxification and immune-regulating systems. When the gut is compromised, the skin often becomes the secondary site of inflammation.

The gastrointestinal tract is lined with a mucosal barrier that protects against pathogens, toxins, and undigested food particles. When that barrier is damaged, a condition often referred to as increased intestinal permeability or "leaky gut," toxins and inflammatory compounds can enter the bloodstream and trigger systemic immune responses. These inflammatory signals can circulate to the skin, contributing to conditions such as acne, eczema, psoriasis, and chronic hives.

Disruptions in the gut microbiome, the diverse population of bacteria and other microbes that inhabit the digestive tract, can also impact the skin. A healthy gut flora produces short-chain fatty acids and metabolites that regulate inflammation, support immune tolerance, and influence hormone levels. An imbalanced gut microbiome, also known as dysbiosis, can promote chronic inflammation, oxidative stress, and hormonal imbalances that manifest visibly on the skin.

Emerging studies, including De Pessemier et al. (2021), have shown that certain strains of beneficial gut bacteria are associated with healthier skin and lower rates of inflammatory skin conditions. Conversely, a reduced microbial diversity in the gut is correlated with more severe dermatological symptoms. There is also growing evidence that topical absorption of harmful chemicals, especially endocrine disruptors found in personal care products, can alter the gut microbiota indirectly by influencing systemic immune and metabolic pathways.

Furthermore, poor gut function impairs the body's ability to detoxify. If the liver, kidneys, or intestinal tract cannot properly eliminate toxins, those compounds may be pushed out through the skin, a backup route that can lead to breakouts, rashes, or flare-ups.

In this sense, the skin is often the body's last line of defense, signaling that internal systems are under strain.

To support both gut and skin health, it is essential to reduce external exposures to irritants while also rebuilding the gut from the inside. This may include nutrient-dense foods, fermented vegetables, bone broth, and targeted probiotics, alongside the removal of processed foods and synthetic chemical exposures from body care routines.

The path to clear, resilient skin often begins in the gut. Understanding this dynamic gives individuals a broader framework for healing that extends beyond surface-level solutions and invites a more holistic, integrated approach to wellness.

Simplifying for Healing

Healing is not about adding more. It is about subtracting what does not serve. Many people experience dramatic improvements in their skin by removing rather than adding.

Start by eliminating:

- Products with added fragrance or parfum

- Items with long, synthetic-heavy ingredient lists

- Anything with known EDCs such as parabens, phthalates, and oxybenzone

- Harsh exfoliants, peels, and drying treatments

Replace with:

- Single-ingredient, bio-compatible moisturizers like tallow or emu oil

- Non-nano, mineral-based sunscreens

- Cleansers made with raw honey, oils, or gentle saltwater

The goal is to rebuild the skin's microbiome and barrier function, both of which play critical roles in immune response and moisture retention. Real healing does not come from masking symptoms. It comes from restoring balance.

In the next chapter, we will explore the rise of the "natural" and "clean beauty" movements. While these were originally created in response to toxic mainstream products, they have become industries in their own right. We will examine how greenwashing, unregulated claims, and trendy branding continue to mislead consumers who are simply trying to make safer choices.

When we think of skincare, we think of radiance. Glow. Clarity. But more and more people-especially women-are waking up to faces that feel inflamed, irritated, and reactive. Despite spending hundreds or even thousands of dollars on products, the skin doesn't get healthier. It gets angrier.

The irony? Many of the very products promising transformation are triggering the issues they claim to fix.

In the next chapter, we'll explore how the "natural" and "clean beauty" movements tried to fix this crisis-but often became part of the problem. We'll break down how greenwashing sells safety while still sneaking in hidden dangers.

CHAPTER 6:

The "Natural" Lie

As public awareness of toxic ingredients began to grow, a new trend emerged to soothe consumer anxiety: "clean beauty." Shelves filled with green labels, kraft paper packaging, and words like "pure," "eco," and "natural." It felt like a cultural shift. It felt like the industry had finally listened. But for many companies, clean beauty was never a commitment to safer products. It was a clever pivot in branding, a new aesthetic overlay placed atop the same old formulas.

Greenwashing 101

The term "greenwashing" was first coined in the 1980s to describe the misleading practice of portraying environmentally harmful practices as eco-conscious. In the beauty industry, this tactic evolved into a form of marketing deception that capitalizes on consumer fears while offering the illusion of health and sustainability. It has become a strategy of optics rather than substance.

Many companies engage in greenwashing by using earth-toned packaging, buzzwords like "eco," "clean," or "natural," and nature-themed imagery such as leaves or water droplets. These visual cues suggest purity and health, but they are rarely backed by regulatory standards or scientific transparency.

In many cases, products that are marketed as "natural" or "green" still contain synthetic preservatives like phenoxyethanol, petroleum-based emollients, and even undisclosed fragrance blends that may harbor phthalates or allergens. Highlighting a single botanical extract like aloe vera or chamomile often distracts consumers from more concerning ingredients buried in the label. A product can feature one organic oil and still include carcinogens, hormone disruptors, and allergens.

Moreover, many brands engage in "ingredient tokenism" using a minute quantity of a trendy or recognizable natural ingredient to justify broad marketing claims. This tactic gives consumers the sense that the product is safe or plant-based, when in fact the majority of its formulation remains chemically conventional. These claims are further reinforced through influencer marketing and vague product promises, which increase perceived trustworthiness without providing true safety or transparency.

According to a 2022 report by the Environmental Working Group (EWG), over 60 percent of personal care products marketed with health-forward claims still contain at least one ingredient flagged as a potential hazard. Without legally enforceable definitions for terms like "clean," "green," or "natural," brands are free to define them as they see fit. This lack of standardization creates confusion and makes it nearly impossible for well-meaning consumers to discern marketing from meaningful reform.

In essence, greenwashing in cosmetics is not simply deceptive, it actively undermines the health-first intentions of consumers by creating a false sense of safety. It transforms consumer empowerment into a marketing strategy, while the burden of risk remains with the individual.

A true clean product is not just free from synthetics. It is transparent, simple, and designed to support biology, not exploit trends. The following sections will break down why not all natural ingredients are inherently safe and how this marketing playbook continues to shape purchasing behavior and public perception.

Greenwashing is the practice of using environmental or health-conscious marketing to mask harmful or unchanged practices. In cosmetics, it often looks like:

- Packaging that mimics homemade or artisanal products

- Claims like "non-toxic," "chemical-free," or "natural," none of which are legally defined

- Highlighting one or two plant-based ingredients while the rest of the formula still contains synthetic preservatives, allergens, or known endocrine disruptors

According to the Environmental Working Group (EWG), there are no federal regulations around the terms "natural," "clean," or "green" in cosmetics. This means a company can label a product "natural" even if 90 percent of its formulation contains petrochemicals or synthetic fragrance compounds (EWG, 2022).

These marketing terms are not safety certifications. They are unregulated claims designed to meet the rising demand for healthier products without requiring meaningful reformulation. In essence, greenwashing sells comfort, not safety.

When "Natural" Isn't Safer

There is a persistent and misleading assumption in the wellness and beauty world that if something is labeled "natural," it must be safe. This belief is not only scientifically unfounded, but potentially dangerous. While many natural ingredients offer therapeutic benefits, others are highly bioactive, unstable, or sensitizing to the skin. And in the context of cosmetic formulations, even a beneficial substance can become problematic when used at inappropriate concentrations, applied over time, or mixed with other actives.

Consider essential oils. While lavender and tea tree oils are often marketed as gentle and healing, research shows that these oils contain compounds that can act as endocrine disruptors. A study by Henley et al. (2007) published in the New England Journal of Medicine found that repeated topical exposure to these oils may be linked to prepubertal gynecomastia (breast tissue development) in boys, suggesting hormone-altering effects.

Similarly, citrus oils such as bergamot or lemon can cause phototoxic reactions when applied to the skin before sun exposure. The result can be long-lasting hyperpigmentation, increased photosensitivity, or even chemical burns. These oils are widely used in "natural" skincare despite limited public knowledge about these risks.

Plant-based preservatives like potassium sorbate or benzyl alcohol are often added to "green" beauty products to extend shelf life. While these alternatives are less controversial than formaldehyde releasers, they can still cause irritation, especially in individuals with sensitive or reactive skin. Moreover, they are rarely tested in combination with other ingredients, leaving users vulnerable to cumulative sensitization.

Another common group of ingredients are coconut-derived surfactants, such as sodium coco-sulfate or cocamidopropyl betaine. These compounds are often marketed as gentler alternatives to sodium lauryl sulfate. Yet they still function as foaming agents and can be harsh on the skin's lipid barrier, especially with daily use.

Without full transparency and robust safety testing, even the most promising plant-based ingredients can lead to adverse outcomes. The myth that "natural" equals non-toxic has allowed many poorly formulated products to flood the market under the guise of clean living. These products may be free from parabens or phthalates, but that does not guarantee they are safe, effective, or compatible with your skin's unique biology.

In truth, natural ingredients deserve the same level of scrutiny as their synthetic counterparts. Responsible formulation requires more than a return to nature, it demands scientific literacy, integrity in sourcing, and a commitment to long-term safety over short-term trends.

The Role of Influencers

Social media influencers have become some of the most powerful marketing forces in the modern beauty landscape. Their rise coincided perfectly with the emergence of the clean beauty trend.

As trust in large corporations began to erode, consumers turned to peer-like voices, often women who appeared relatable, authentic, and aligned with wellness values. Brands capitalized on this cultural shift by sending free product packages, offering affiliate codes, and paying influencers to promote new "natural" or "clean" launches.

The appeal of these influencers is undeniable. They speak casually from their bathrooms, film "get ready with me" routines, and share personal skin stories. This style of communication feels honest and trustworthy. But many of these individuals lack any formal education in dermatology, cosmetic chemistry, or toxicology. Without scientific literacy, influencers may repeat marketing claims without vetting the product formulations themselves.

As a result, millions of followers have unknowingly replaced one set of problematic products with another. Many abandoned synthetics like parabens or synthetic fragrance only to embrace essential oil-heavy products or antioxidant-rich serums that, while labeled clean, still disrupted their skin barrier or hormonal balance. The problem is not always in what is used, but in the assumption that these influencers are speaking from an informed, evidence-based foundation.

For example, some popular influencers have recommended applying undiluted essential oils directly to the skin, something even trained aromatherapists strongly caution against. Others promote layering multiple active botanicals without understanding pH balance, skin tolerance, or product incompatibilities. This kind of guidance, while well-intentioned, can contribute to barrier damage, irritation, or long-term sensitivity.

It is worth noting that some influencers are doing important work. A growing number of content creators with science backgrounds are using their platforms to demystify formulation claims, debunk greenwashing, and advocate for ingredient transparency. But their voices are often drowned out by more glamorous, monetized content that reinforces quick fixes, aesthetic minimalism, or overconsumption of trendy natural products.

In short, the influencer economy has amplified both awareness and confusion. It has helped elevate concerns about toxicity but has also created new pathways for misinformation and poorly formulated alternatives to thrive. As we navigate the clean beauty space, it is essential to follow educators who prioritize evidence, nuance, and transparency, not just aesthetics, virality, or sponsorships.

Where Clean Beauty Gets It Right

Despite its flaws, the clean beauty movement has prompted important conversations about ingredient transparency, ethical sourcing, and consumer empowerment. Some companies have responded to consumer demand with true integrity.

Brands that prioritize genuine safety tend to:

- Use short, understandable ingredient lists

- Provide full ingredient transparency

- Invest in third-party certifications like EWG Verified, Made Safe, or Leaping Bunny

- Prioritize microbiome health and barrier-supportive formulations

These companies often operate with smaller margins and face stricter scrutiny, but they are helping to set a new standard. The best among them embrace education, inviting consumers to learn about formulation science rather than simply selling aesthetic minimalism.

How to Spot the Real Thing

Navigating clean beauty requires discernment. Consider the following when evaluating a product:

1. Is the full ingredient list disclosed, including fragrance components? Transparency is non-negotiable.

2. Are the product's claims supported by certifications or evidence-based testing? Buzzwords are meaningless without accountability.

3. Does the brand educate about its sourcing and safety standards? Or does it rely on green fonts and nature imagery?

4. Are the ingredients necessary, or are they chosen to ride a marketing trend? The simplest routines are often the most effective.

Ancestral skincare ingredients tend to be safe and effective precisely because they are time-tested. Tallow, honey, clay, salt, and rendered fats have been used for centuries across cultures. They are biologically compatible with human skin, and they do not require synthetic modification to be effective.

True skin health does not require exotic extracts or trendy packaging. It requires consistency, simplicity, and formulations that respect the skin's natural biology.

In the next chapter, we'll shift focus from critique to action. You'll learn how to detox your beauty routine, audit your products, and rebuild a personal care ritual that honors your health and your body's wisdom.

CHAPTER 7:

The Mirror Mindset Detox

You've made it this far, and if you're here, it means you're ready to do something about it. Awareness is the first step. But action is where change really happens.

A mirror mindset detox is not just about throwing away a few products. It's about rewriting your relationship with beauty, reclaiming your body's authority, and building new rituals that support, not sabotage your health. This isn't a trend. This is a return.

Step 1: The Inventory Audit

Before you can make changes, you have to know what you're working with. Empty out your drawers, shelves, bags, and bathroom cabinets. Lay everything out.

Create three piles:

- Keep (Clean & Trusted)

- Question (Needs Ingredient Review)

- Discard (Toxic, Expired, or Unnecessary)

Use tools like the Environmental Working Group's Skin Deep Database or the Think Dirty app to check ingredient safety. Prioritize products used daily; like moisturizers, foundation, and deodorant, because these contribute the most to toxic load.

Ask of each item:

- Is this necessary?

- Is this safe?

- Is this serving my skin or covering a problem?

Step 2: Understanding Your Skin's Natural Needs

Your skin has innate intelligence. It produces oils, sheds dead cells, responds to climate, and adjusts to stress. Most modern products work *against* this process instead of with it.

You don't need a 12-step routine. You need:

- Gentle cleansing

- Occasional exfoliation (natural acids or honey)

- Nourishing moisture (animal-based fats, olive oil, or jojoba)

- Sun exposure in moderation

By over-cleansing, over-exfoliating, and layering synthetic ingredients, we disrupt the skin's barrier and confuse its natural rhythm. Simplicity restores balance.

Step 3: Swap Smart, Not Fast

Detoxing your beauty products doesn't have to happen overnight. In fact, slow, mindful transitions tend to be more sustainable. Start with the highest-impact categories:

High-Priority Swaps:

1. Deodorant – Conventional antiperspirants often contain aluminum and synthetic fragrance. Try magnesium-based, baking soda-free formulas or mineral sprays.

2. Moisturizer – Replace chemical-laden lotions with tallow balm, shea butter, or cold-pressed oils.

3. Foundation & Concealer – Many contain silicone, petroleum byproducts, and parabens. Look for mineral-based alternatives with simple formulas.

4. Lip products – Lipsticks are often ingested in small amounts. Avoid synthetic dyes, fragrance, and lead contamination.

Optional-But-Helpful Swaps:

- Shampoo and conditioner (avoid sulfates and artificial fragrance)

- Sunscreen (choose non-nano zinc oxide over chemical filters)

- Mascara (look for wax-based, fragrance-free options)

Each swap is a vote for your long-term health. Each product you don't repurchase is a disruption in a broken system, and a decision that puts money back in your pocket. Simplifying your routine doesn't just support your biology, it also reduces financial stress. Fewer products, used more intentionally, means less waste and more freedom.

Step 4: Embrace Ancestral Rituals

The solutions to vibrant, healthy skin are not innovations, they are rediscoveries. Long before commercial skincare existed, ancestral cultures thrived using ingredients sourced directly from their ecosystems. These were not fads. They were rituals rooted in observation, seasonality, and respect for the body's natural processes.

Ancestral skincare is about relationship. Relationship to land, to body, to simplicity. And it carries with it an intuitive intelligence that modern products often ignore in favor of aggressive, one-size-fits-all formulas.

- Tallow balm: Rendered from grass-fed beef fat, tallow closely mimics the fatty acid profile of human skin. It is rich in fat-soluble vitamins A, D, E, and K—nutrients essential for skin regeneration, elasticity, and barrier integrity. Used daily, it can help restore moisture balance, soothe inflammation, and support the microbiome without clogging pores.

- Raw honey: Known for its antimicrobial and humectant properties, raw honey supports wound healing, acne-prone skin, and hydration. Its low pH helps maintain the skin's acid mantle, while enzymes and trace minerals offer nourishment.

- Clay masks: Bentonite and French green clay have been used for centuries to detoxify the skin. Rich in minerals, these clays draw out impurities, support lymphatic drainage, and help remineralize the skin—particularly when blended with hydrosols or apple cider vinegar.

- Apple cider vinegar (ACV): Diluted ACV works as a gentle, pH-balancing toner that supports the skin's natural acidity, helps prevent bacterial overgrowth, and can reduce irritation when used mindfully.

These ingredients are not only effective but economical. A small jar of tallow balm can last for months. A teaspoon of honey becomes a mask. A splash of vinegar becomes a toner. These aren't just skin treatments, they're invitations to slow down, to tend, to ritualize.

Unlike commercial products that often encourage daily overuse, ancestral ingredients encourage restraint. You use what you need and nothing more. This minimalism is not only more supportive of the skin, it's more sustainable for the planet and for your wallet.

Reclaiming ancestral care is about more than what you put on your face. It's a cultural and physiological reset. It tells your nervous system, "You are safe now. You are cared for."

In a world that profits from your insecurity, these ancestral rituals are acts of quiet rebellion, and deep remembrance.

Step 5: Rebuild Ritual Without Perfectionism

Let go of the idea that you need to "fix" your skin. Detoxing is not a punishment. It's a return to partnership with your body, your biology, and your own instincts.

Replace anxiety with care:

- Massage your face with oil instead of scrubbing it raw.

- Apply tallow balm at night as a ritual of nourishment.

- Let your skin breathe during the day, without layers of coverage.

- Use scent sparingly, intentionally, if at all.

This is not about doing everything perfectly. This is about choosing what's aligned with truth.

What to Expect When You Detox

When you begin removing toxic products and replacing them with simpler, ancestral alternatives, your body responds. This is a healing process, but it is not always linear, and it does not always look pretty.

The skin, being an organ of elimination, often reflects what the body is processing internally. As you phase out conventional products, many of which include steroids, hormone-mimicking preservatives, or occlusive agents like silicones, your skin may go through a transition period. This phase is sometimes referred to as "skin purging," but what it really represents is recalibration.

You may experience:

- Increased breakouts, especially if you previously used pore-blocking or antibiotic-based products

- Temporary dryness or flaking as your skin adjusts oil production and barrier function

- Sensitivity to sun, wind, or even water as your acid mantle heals and strengthens

- Shifts in texture or tone as dead skin layers are shed and replaced

These symptoms are not regressions. They are communications. Your body is asking for patience, nourishment, and consistency, not another round of aggressive treatments.

Internally, detoxing may stir up other responses as well, such as fatigue, mild headaches, or temporary digestive changes. This is especially true if you're pairing your skincare detox with dietary shifts or removing major sources of endocrine disruption. Supporting your liver and lymphatic system through hydration, mineral-rich broths, gentle movement, and sleep will help your body process these shifts more smoothly.

Track your progress. Write down what you're using, how your skin is responding, how you're feeling emotionally. Detox is not just a surface change it often brings up old insecurities, doubts, or stories we've attached to appearance. Let them come up. Witness them without judgment. And return to your ritual.

With consistency, most people notice improvement in barrier health, inflammation reduction, and overall radiance within a few weeks to a few months. The timeline varies, but the direction is always toward deeper harmony.

What you are doing is not cosmetic. It is biological, psychological, and ancestral. Give it time to root..

Your Gut: The Hidden Partner in Skin Detox

While this chapter focuses on external products and skin health, it's important to recognize that detox is a full-body process, and your gut is central to it. The gut and the skin are deeply connected through the immune system, hormonal pathways, and detoxification channels. If your gut is inflamed, imbalanced, or overburdened, the skin will often express that internal imbalance.

When you detox your skincare, your body begins offloading stored toxins. These must be metabolized and eliminated primarily through the liver and the digestive tract. If your gut is not functioning optimally, due to leaky gut, dysbiosis, or poor bile flow those toxins may recirculate, triggering breakouts, rashes, or inflammation that shows up on your face.

To support your gut during this transition:

- Focus on nutrient density with a carnivore or low-carb ancestral diet, rich in ruminant animal fats and proteins

- Consume collagen-rich bone broth to help seal and nourish the gut lining

- Prioritize organs, pasture-raised meat, and electrolyte balance for optimal digestion and detox support

- Eliminate ultra-processed foods, seed oils, and fiber-heavy plant matter that can irritate the gut lining in sensitive individuals

Contrary to mainstream advice, fiber is not digestible by the human body. While it is often promoted for digestive health, especially in conventional nutrition circles, the reality is that humans lack the enzymes necessary to break down fiber. Instead of nourishing the gut, excessive fiber intake can ferment in the digestive tract, leading to bloating, irritation, or exacerbated leaky gut symptoms, particularly in those with compromised gut health. From an ancestral perspective, early human diets prioritized nutrient-dense animal foods that require minimal digestive effort while delivering maximum bioavailability. An animal-based approach offers deep cellular repair, gut lining restoration, and hormonal support without the digestive burden posed by indigestible plant fibers.

Your skin will reflect the clarity of your inner terrain. Healing is more than what you remove from your bathroom shelf, it's also what you repair within. Restoring the gut supports hormone balance, detoxification, and immune resilience, all of which translate to visible improvements in skin health.

This is not about perfection. It's about partnership. Partner with your body, your gut, your skin. Together, they know how to restore.

Why This Matters

Every product you eliminate, every ingredient you research, every ancestral ritual you reclaim, it's a radical act of health sovereignty.

You're not just detoxing your mirror mindset. You're detoxing decades of messaging that told you your skin, your face, your body needed constant improvement.

In the next chapter, we'll explore how redefining beauty on your own terms becomes an act of rebellion and resilience. Aging becomes a gift. Strength becomes the new glow. And beauty becomes something you no longer chase, but *inhabit*.

CHAPTER 8:

The Beauty Rebellion

There comes a moment in every transformation when the internal shift becomes visible, not on the skin, but in the eyes. A sense of peace. Of ownership. Of finally stepping out of the chase and into something deeper, something rooted in truth and no longer dictated by marketing metrics or cultural illusions.

This is the beauty rebellion.

Not loud. Not angry. But calm, confident, and sovereign. A quiet refusal to participate in a system that profits from our self-doubt. A deliberate return to what is real, ancestral, and biologically sound.

Redefining Beauty for Yourself

What if beauty wasn't something to earn or maintain, but something to notice and honor? What if your crow's feet were proof of laughter? Your stretch marks, a record of growth? What if the face you see in the mirror didn't need contouring or concealing to be worthy of care?

Real beauty has nothing to do with flawlessness. It has everything to do with presence, energy, and vitality. These come from within, and they radiate when the body is nourished, the mind is grounded, and the spirit is free from shame.

And here's a truth that rarely gets voiced: most men, especially those seeking real connection, are not drawn to the overdone, filtered, or surgically altered version of beauty promoted by mainstream media. They are not looking for a perfectly sculpted face or a masked appearance. They are drawn to authenticity. To warmth. To skin that moves, to faces that age, to expressions that reflect a full and vibrant life, a real, natural woman.

Time and again, men report that they prefer the "natural" look, not because it is more appealing in a conventional sense, but because it feels real, trustworthy, and inviting. The fake lashes, contoured jawlines, and glassy skin often create distance, not intimacy. When you stop altering your appearance to meet a cultural fantasy, you step into a version of yourself that feels grounded and magnetic, not because of how you look, but because of how you feel in your skin.

The rebellion begins with redefining what beauty means to you:

- Is it about being seen? Or being *whole*?

- Is it about control? Or collaboration with your body?

- Is it about looking younger? Or living with more vitality?

Let these questions guide your choices. Let them strip away every external voice that told you how you *should* look.

Living Outside the Metrics

In a world obsessed with before-and-after photos, likes, filters, and constant digital comparison, choosing not to engage is nothing short of radical. We are conditioned to seek validation through external feedback. The dopamine rush of a "like" or a flattering comment has been engineered to keep us dependent on outside approval. But living outside these metrics is where true freedom begins.

This isn't about disappearing or rejecting beauty altogether. It's about choosing a different metric, your own sense of vitality, peace, and embodied presence. It's about showing up for yourself on your terms.

Living outside the metrics means:

- Wearing less makeup, or none at all, and noticing how your nervous system responds to being seen naturally.

- Letting your hair gray, grow wild, or be what it is without apology or performance.

- Choosing skincare because it supports your health, not because it promises to "erase" or "tighten."

- Prioritizing nervous system regulation over image management. Slowing down. Eating slowly. Walking barefoot. Looking people in the eyes without wondering what they see back.

This is a bold choice in a society that profits from your dissatisfaction. Stepping out of the comparison economy isn't passive; it's active resistance. It takes courage to be visible in your natural state, especially in spaces where filters and fine-tuned lighting dominate perception.

And here's the truth: when you begin to disconnect from the metrics, your inner voice gets louder. You'll begin to notice what actually feels good in your body, what rituals restore you, what foods give you clarity and strength. You'll stop outsourcing your self-worth to algorithms and influencers.

You don't owe anyone a polished face. Not your employer, not your online following, not even your partner. What you owe yourself is consistency, nourishment, and integrity. You owe yourself the right to opt out without explanation, to live unmeasured, and to reclaim your time, attention, and inner quiet.

This is not about disappearing. It's about becoming visible in a new way, on your own terms.

Raising the Next Generation Differently

This rebellion isn't just for us, it is for those who are watching, absorbing, and mimicking our every move. Children are born with no innate judgment about their appearance, but from a young age they are exposed to messaging that ties their worth to how they look. This happens subtly and persistently, through advertising, screen time, peer comparison, and yes, even in the way adults talk about their own bodies.

Psychologists have long observed that children internalize standards of beauty early. Research shows that by age three, children begin to prefer certain body types based on what they see represented in media. By age six, girls already express a desire to be thinner, and by adolescence, body dissatisfaction becomes a leading contributor to anxiety, low self-esteem, and disordered eating. This is not coincidence, it is cultural conditioning.

The good news is that this pattern can be interrupted. Children learn most through modeling. When we choose authenticity, self-respect, and nourishment over performance, they absorb that too.

You can rewire the narrative they inherit:

- Speak kindly about your body in their presence, even on the hard days.

- Avoid commenting on others' bodies, weight, or aging. Praise function over form.

- Normalize care as a form of respect, not correction or punishment.

- Teach them to question advertising and understand that marketing plays on fear, not fact.

- Affirm that their value comes from who they are, not what they look like.

Imagine a child growing up believing their body is already enough. That their reflection is not a problem to solve. That they are allowed to age, to change, and to take up space without apology. That is the real revolution, and it begins at home.

Community Over Competition

The modern beauty industry thrives on division. It pits women against one another in a silent arms race of perfection. But competition dissolves in the presence of genuine connection.

One of the most powerful antidotes to comparison culture is authentic female friendship. Research in psychology consistently shows that strong social bonds, particularly among women, are essential to emotional resilience, stress reduction, and even longevity. Girlfriends offer something deeper than camaraderie. They offer reflection. When you are seen and accepted by women who know your story and support your truth, you are less vulnerable to the narratives that tell you you're not enough.

Female friendships support regulation of the nervous system through co-regulation: a process where shared presence, eye contact, and empathetic listening help the body feel safe. These relationships also provide a buffer against the self-doubt that arises in beauty-saturated spaces. When your close circle values laughter, nourishment, creativity, and care over appearance, it becomes easier to release the pressure to perform.

And when women support each other, something bigger shifts. We step out of silent competition and into collective reclamation.

Build communities rooted in encouragement, truth, and healing:

- Compliment qualities of presence, confidence, and creativity, not just aesthetics.

- Share ancestral recipes, healing protocols, and skin rituals.

- Support others stepping away from the hamster wheel of self-optimization.

- Prioritize friendship as a wellness tool, not an afterthought.

When we create spaces where people are safe to be unfiltered, unedited, and alive, we shift the cultural narrative. The rebellion multiplies in the community. modern beauty industry thrives on division. It pits women against one another in a silent arms race of perfection. But competition dissolves in the presence of genuine connection.

Beauty as Aliveness

When we stop trying to fix ourselves, what emerges is something honest and magnetic. A beauty that is not still, frozen, or filtered, but alive.

Aliveness looks like:

- Cheeks flushed from sun, movement, or laughter

- Eyes lit with curiosity, rest, and purpose

- Skin marked by time, touched by care, and nourished from within

- Posture that speaks of self-respect, not self-monitoring

This glow cannot be bought or bottled. It is the result of honoring your body, feeding it species-appropriate food, letting it move, and giving it rest. It is remembering what it feels like to live in your skin without apology.

You don't need fixing. You need nourishment. You need truth. You need to come home to yourself.

In the next chapter, we'll build your long-term support system, tools and strategies to sustain your health and radiance from the inside out. Because rebellion begins with a spark, but it's consistency that carries it forward.

CHAPTER 9:

Building Your Clean Living Toolkit

Rebellion without structure burns out fast. The fire starts with awareness, but it's sustained by routine, by community, and by tools that help you live your truth every single day.

This chapter is about support. Because healing doesn't happen in isolation, and detoxing your mirror mindset is just the beginning. Real change sticks when it integrates into your daily rhythm.

Your Skin is an Ecosystem

Your skin is alive. It houses bacteria, yeast, sebum, sweat, and cells that constantly renew. It interacts with your nervous system, your gut, your lymph, and your immune response. A healthy skin ecosystem doesn't just "look good," it *functions* well.

Supporting that ecosystem means giving it:

- Clean nourishment (internally and externally)

- Time to heal

- Products that don't interfere with its natural processes

Let's build your toolkit around that.

Everyday Essentials

You don't need 20 products. You need a few, well-chosen allies. Here's a simple baseline toolkit, with a clear explanation for each:

Cleanser

- Oil cleansing (jojoba, tallow, olive oil) – These natural oils dissolve sebum, makeup, and dirt without stripping the skin's natural barrier. Unlike harsh soaps, they preserve the microbiome and maintain hydration.

- Raw honey or kefir masks – Raw honey is naturally antimicrobial and soothing, while kefir introduces probiotics and enzymes to help balance inflammation and support the skin's natural defenses.

Moisturizer

- Tallow balm – Rich in bioavailable vitamins A, D, E, and K, tallow mimics the skin's natural oils. It deeply nourishes without clogging pores and supports skin elasticity and healing.

- Emu oil or beef suet balm – These ancestral fats are high in omega-3s and skin-penetrating lipids that restore compromised barriers and soothe inflamed or dry skin.

Toner (Optional)

- Apple cider vinegar diluted 1:3 with filtered water – Balances skin pH, reduces bacteria, and supports the acid mantle. Its mild astringent properties tighten pores and refresh skin tone.

- Hydrosols (rose, lavender, chamomile) – Plant-based aromatic waters offer gentle toning, hydration, and anti-inflammatory support without disrupting the skin barrier.

Sun Protection

- Eliminate seed oils from your diet – Seed oils like canola, soybean, and sunflower are high in omega-6 polyunsaturated fats. These fats integrate into your cell membranes and increase your susceptibility to oxidative damage. When consumed regularly, they may contribute to a higher risk of sunburn and accelerated aging due to lipid peroxidation in skin tissues.

- Avoid wearing sunglasses during early morning sun exposure – Light entering through the eyes helps regulate your circadian rhythm and signals your body to produce melanin, the skin's natural sun protection. Blocking natural light with sunglasses, especially first thing in the day, can interfere with hormonal balance, sleep quality, and your skin's resilience to sunlight.

- Wide-brim hat, mineral-based zinc sunscreen – Physical sun barriers prevent overexposure without interfering with vitamin D synthesis. Zinc oxide offers broad-spectrum protection without the hormone-disrupting chemicals found in many conventional sunscreens.

- Early morning sun exposure – Gradual exposure to sunlight builds melanin and supports your circadian rhythm, helping your skin naturally become more resilient to UV damage.

Makeup (if you choose to wear it)

- Mineral-based powders – Free from fillers, dyes, and preservatives, these offer light coverage without clogging pores or irritating sensitive skin.

- Cream-based blush/lip tint with clean ingredients – Look for products with tallow, beeswax, or castor oil bases. These nourish while adding natural color.

- Avoid products with "fragrance," PEGs, silicones, parabens, and synthetic dyes – These additives can disrupt hormones, clog pores, or irritate skin over time.

Internal Allies

Because beauty is an inside job, your skin will reflect the health of your digestion, hormones, and immune system. Consider integrating:

- Bone broth – Rich in collagen, glycine, and minerals that support gut repair, skin elasticity, and detoxification.

- Beef liver – Nature's multivitamin, loaded with fat-soluble nutrients that support skin regeneration, hormonal balance, and immune function.

- Raw dairy (if tolerated) – High in enzymes, fat-soluble vitamins, and probiotics. Supports hydration, skin structure, and microbiome diversity.

- Magnesium – Essential for over 300 biochemical processes, including skin repair, hormone regulation, and nervous system balance.

- Mineral-rich salts – Support adrenal function, hydration, and cellular communication. Unrefined sea salt and Himalayan salt contain trace minerals that modern diets often lack.

Focus on nutrient density over supplements. Eat food your ancestors would recognize. Simpler is better.

Non-Toxic Living Beyond the Mirror

The skin doesn't stop at your face. Neither should your detox. Clean living expands into your home, your air, your water, and your sensory environment. These changes may seem small, but their cumulative impact is profound, and they lay the groundwork for deeper transformation that we'll explore more fully in a future book focused on the ancestral home and environment. For now, this is where to begin:

Laundry

- Swap synthetic detergents for fragrance-free or soap-based alternatives – Conventional detergents often leave chemical residues that irritate skin.

- Use wool dryer balls with optional essential oils – Reduce static and soften fabric naturally without artificial fragrances.

Home Cleaning

- Vinegar, castile soap, baking soda, and water – These ingredients clean effectively without leaving behind harmful residues.

- Avoid "antibacterial" sprays and wipes – These often contain triclosan or quaternary ammonium compounds that disrupt hormones and damage microbiota.

Water

- Invest in a quality shower filter – Chlorine and fluoride can irritate skin, disrupt microbiota, and interfere with thyroid function.

- Drink filtered water with added minerals – Stay hydrated with clean water. Avoid plastics, which may leach estrogenic compounds into your drinking water.

Air

- Open windows – Natural airflow reduces indoor toxin accumulation.

- Add houseplants – Certain plants like peace lilies and snake plants filter indoor air.

- Consider a HEPA filter if needed – Especially important in urban or industrial areas.

Habits That Heal

More than any product, your lifestyle determines how your skin behaves. A clean routine is only as effective as the habits that support it:

- Sleep deeply – Prioritize 8–9 hours of restorative sleep. During sleep, your body enters critical repair cycles where cellular regeneration peaks, skin detoxification ramps up, and hormone balance is restored. Chronic sleep deprivation disrupts cortisol rhythms and reduces collagen production, both of which accelerate aging and inflammation.

- Move daily – Support lymphatic drainage and circulation. Gentle movement keeps blood flowing, oxygenates tissues, and improves detoxification. Daily yoga or stretching promotes flexibility, stimulates fascia and lymph flow, and helps release stored tension in the body. These movements also support joint health and activate the parasympathetic nervous system, which is essential for recovery, hormonal regulation, and a sense of embodied calm.

- Sweat – Sweat through saunas, hot baths, or physical activity to eliminate stored toxins like heavy metals, phthalates, and BPA. Sweating also enhances mitochondrial function, improves insulin sensitivity, and supports skin clarity by clearing congested pores and promoting turnover.

- Dry brush and cold rinse – Dry brushing boosts circulation and exfoliation by stimulating surface blood flow and encouraging lymph movement. Follow it with a cold rinse to tighten pores, invigorate the skin, and tone the vagus nerve—supporting a regulated nervous system and enhanced immune function.

- Grounding – Barefoot contact with natural surfaces like grass, soil, or sand has been shown to reduce inflammation, lower cortisol, and rebalance circadian rhythms. Grounding restores electrical homeostasis in the body, supporting deeper sleep, calmer moods, and visible improvements in skin texture.

These ancestral habits restore nervous system balance, reduce inflammation, and bring clarity to the skin, and to your life. They are low-cost, high-impact rituals that reconnect you with the rhythms your biology remembers, even if modern culture has forgotten them.

Making It Stick

The most important part of your toolkit? Consistency. Not perfection. Not panic. Just showing up for yourself every day with small, repeatable care. When you build a rhythm rooted in nourishment and respect, your body responds.

You don't need to obsess. You need to *align*.

In the next chapter, we'll explore how this new way of living connects you with others, and how sharing your story can spark change in your community, your home, and even across generations.

CHAPTER 10:

Community, Culture & Conversation

You weren't meant to do this alone.

Healing, reclaiming, and redefining beauty isn't just a personal journey, it's a cultural shift. And it's one that grows stronger in community. When you speak truth, you give others permission to do the same. When you live differently, visibly, you show what's possible.

This chapter is about connection. Because changing your own habits is powerful, but changing the conversation changes everything.

The Power of Telling Your Story

Your voice has weight. When you share your experience, what led you to detox your mirror mindset, what you discovered, how you felt, you become a mirror for others. Not a guru. Not a guide. A witness. You carry proof that another way is not only possible, it is already unfolding.

In a world where beauty culture thrives on silence and comparison, personal storytelling breaks the spell. It doesn't just educate, it liberates. Each time you name what you've walked through, you help someone else locate their own voice. And in doing so, you shift the collective conversation.

We need more witnesses. More people willing to say:

- "I was exhausted by beauty culture."

- "I thought I was broken, but I wasn't."

- "This is what helped me heal."

- "This is how I reclaimed my body."

- "This is what changed when I stopped apologizing."

Stories disarm. They reach beyond data and tap into memory, emotion, and identity. They humanize. They ground us. They make healing feel less abstract and more embodied.

You can tell your story over coffee, in your journal, on a walk, through a podcast, in a social media post, or even in silence, by showing up differently. Storytelling doesn't require a platform. It requires presence.

Even if you don't think anyone is listening, someone always is. And the person most transformed might be you.

Culture Begins at Home

It's easy to look at media and think culture is created by celebrities or ad agencies. But the truth is, culture is built one conversation at a time, in kitchens, in car rides, in the quiet moments before bedtime. And for better or worse, some of the deepest programming about beauty and worth happens in the home.

Children are always watching. They absorb not just what we say about them, but how we speak about ourselves. If they hear us critiquing our wrinkles, apologizing for going makeup-free, or obsessing over our weight, they internalize those patterns. If they see us nourishing ourselves with respect, celebrating the aging process, and opting out of beauty shame, they learn to do the same.

Start where you are:

- Model makeup-free days in your home and speak positively about your bare face.

- Compliment others for their energy, creativity, or kindness, not their appearance.

- Talk to your children about what ads are really selling and why the beauty standard changes so often.

- Ask questions like: "How does this make you feel?" instead of "Do I look okay?"

- Normalize ancestral routines like applying tallow together, or oil brushing as a ritual of care rather than correction.

The family bathroom counter is a more powerful cultural arena than you've been led to believe. What happens there, what is said, what is unsaid, echoes into the next generation.

Hosting a "Mirror Mindset" Circle

Want to bring this message to others in a more structured and supportive way? Hosting a "Mirror Mindset" Circle is one of the most powerful ways to deepen your own healing while helping others feel seen. These circles aren't about preaching or presenting, they're about gathering, witnessing, and remembering who we are without the layers of pressure and performance.

You can host a circle in your living room, around a campfire, during a weekly Zoom call, or even inside a group message thread. The point isn't perfection. It's presence. It's creating a container where others feel safe to share without needing to justify, apologize, or hide.

Here's how to begin:

1. Invite 3 to 10 people you trust to show up with openness. These can be friends, family, coworkers, or women from your local community.

2. Choose a focus: read a chapter from this book, watch a documentary, or simply ask a thought-provoking question like, "When did you first feel you weren't enough?"

3. Use a mirror as a prompt: pass it around and ask, "What were you taught to see here, and what do you choose to see now?"

4. Share clean swaps and ancestral rituals: discuss practical tools, favorite products, and mindset shifts that have supported you.

5. Close with a ritual: this could be applying tallow, soaking feet in warm salt water, sitting in silence, or breathing together with one hand on the heart and one on the belly.

You don't need to be an expert. You only need to be honest. These spaces remind us that real transformation doesn't happen on screens, it happens in circles, where the masks come off and the real faces emerge.

Start small. Let the connection grow. You are not just sharing ideas, you're rebuilding culture, like roots, from the ground up.

Building a Better Beauty Culture

What if beauty culture was built on resilience instead of insecurity? What if the standards were:

- Sustainability over speed

- Roots over trends

- Community over comparison

- Wholeness over perfection

You're already doing it. Every clean swap, every honest post, every conversation that breaks the silence, it's laying the bricks for something new.

And here's the beautiful thing: culture doesn't need to be big to be real. You don't need a viral moment. You need consistency, courage, and community.

In the next chapter, we'll explore how to protect what you've built, long-term practices for staying rooted in your values, even when it's hard. Because change is easy to start. Keeping it alive takes heart.

CHAPTER 11:

Staying Rooted

Starting is powerful. But staying rooted, especially in a world that profits off distraction, is sacred work.

This chapter is about longevity. About protecting the clarity you've reclaimed and building a rhythm that supports you for the long haul.

Because there will be pressure. Old voices, new trends, and subtle temptations will whisper: "Just one product," "Just to fix this one thing," "Just to keep up."

But you've already remembered something deeper. Let's keep you anchored in it.

Create a Personal Philosophy

Rules break. Trends shift. But a philosophy, a core set of values can guide your decisions no matter what the beauty industry invents next. It becomes your compass when old habits try to creep back in or when you're tempted to chase the latest "fix."

A personal philosophy gives you language. It grounds your choices in clarity instead of impulse. It helps you pause, question, and come back to yourself, especially when marketing noise is loud or when doubt surfaces in front of the mirror.

This isn't about rigid doctrine. It's about remembering what's true for *you*. What feels nourishing, what aligns with your biology, your ancestry, your integrity.

Write your own skincare (and self-care) philosophy. A few prompts:

- My skin is not a problem to solve. It is...

- I choose products that make me feel...

- I define beauty as...

- My care rituals must support...

- I protect my energy by...

- I reject the belief that...

Revisit this regularly. Let it evolve with you, like a living document. Tape it to your mirror. Keep it in your journal. Make it your quiet declaration of sovereignty in a world that profits from your confusion.

Your philosophy is your anchor. Return to it as often as needed.

Track How You Feel, Not Just How You Look

Photos can be powerful, but they don't always capture the full spectrum of healing. The mirror might show smoother skin or brighter eyes, but it will never fully reflect the deeper shifts that happen beneath the surface. Healing is multidimensional. It affects your energy, mood, mental clarity, and relationship with your body.

Instead of only watching the mirror, track:

- Energy levels – Are you waking with more vitality? Are your afternoon slumps fading?

- Cycle or hormonal shifts – Is your period more regular, less painful, or more intuitive?

- Sleep quality – Are you falling asleep more easily, waking feeling rested, or dreaming more vividly?

- Confidence and self-talk – Are you speaking to yourself with more compassion? Do you notice less internal judgment?

- Skin *feel*, not just appearance – Does your skin feel stronger, calmer, less reactive, or more nourished?

Use a journal, a notes app, or even a daily mood tracker. If you're looking for a supportive and structured way to track your healing journey, consider using *My Carnivore Journal*. It's designed to help you document not only your nutrition but also your mood, skin changes, energy levels, and overall wellness, giving you a clear, tangible record of your progress over time. Check in with yourself weekly or monthly. Ask, "What's changing that I can't see in a photo?"

This is about collecting the kind of data that actually matters. Not numbers. Not before-and-after comparisons. But the lived experience of healing, your capacity to feel good in your body, to move through your day with ease, and to trust yourself again.

The mirror will eventually reflect what you've reclaimed inside. Let how you feel be the guide.

Build Boundaries with Media

The modern beauty industry doesn't just live on shelves, it lives in your feed. And that's by design. Visual exposure is one of the fastest ways to program the brain. Neuroscience shows that the images we take in repeatedly, especially those tied to status, desire, or fear, restructure how we think, feel, and relate to ourselves.

What you see shapes how you see yourself. Studies in cognitive psychology reveal that repeated exposure to digitally altered images can increase anxiety, body dissatisfaction, and even depressive symptoms. For young people, especially girls, curated content on social media can create unrealistic beauty ideals that become internalized long before they're questioned (Fardouly et al., 2015; Tiggemann & Slater, 2014; Perloff, 2014).

To stay rooted in your own truth, you must actively curate your visual and mental environment:

- Curate your social media – Follow people who align with your values, not just aesthetics. Look for creators who share nourishing routines, ancestral wisdom, and honest reflections.

- Mute or unfollow accounts that trigger comparison, consumption, or self-doubt. Your peace is more important than staying "in the loop."

- Take screen sabbaths – Full days or weekends without social media help reset your nervous system and reorient your attention toward real life.

- Use positive input apps – Apps like I Am, Shine, or ThinkUp deliver affirmations and positive self-talk throughout the day. These tools reinforce healthier neural pathways and support emotional resilience.

- Practice mirror affirmations – Say aloud or mentally repeat affirming phrases while looking at yourself: "I am rooted in truth." "My body is wise." "I am enough without fixing." It may feel awkward at first, but over time, these words become anchors.

Your nervous system can't regulate when it's being constantly sold to. Protect your perception. Your internal world is shaped by what your eyes consume. Make it a conscious, nourishing choice.

Anchor in Ritual, Not Reaction

Ritual grounds you. It transforms fleeting moments into meaningful practices. It takes the place of reactivity, which is driven by impulse, and replaces it with rhythm, which is driven by intention.

In a world that encourages us to rush, consume, and compare, ritual invites us to return to the body. To slow down. To reconnect with what is sacred, cyclical, and personal.

Try this:

- Morning: Wash your face with cool water to gently wake the skin and the nervous system. Apply tallow balm with intention, not urgency. Speak one kind truth to yourself. Something simple, like: "I am enough," or "My body knows what to do."

- Night: Oil cleanse slowly to release the day's buildup, both physical and emotional. Breathe deeply, hold a stretch, and exhale the tension you've carried. Take a warm bubble bath to soften the body and mind, using mineral-rich salts or soothing essential oils like lavender. Afterward, use a sleep mask to block ambient light and deepen your rest. Sleeping in full darkness supports melatonin production, cellular repair, and hormonal regulation.

- Weekly: Journal what's working and what's not. Track patterns in your mood, energy, skin texture, and triggers. Take progress photos, not to obsess or compare, but to witness your transformation with perspective and care. Use this check-in not to criticize, but to learn. To listen. Let the visual and emotional reflections work together to remind you of how far you've come.

These moments tether you to what matters. They don't have to be elaborate. They just have to be *yours*. Ritual creates structure where chaos wants to creep in. It becomes a safe container where healing can unfold without pressure.

Over time, your rituals become a form of inner architecture. They hold you steady through seasons of change. They remind you who you are, even when the world tries to tell you otherwise.

Find Accountability That Feels Like Nourishment

Not all community is helpful. Some spaces reinforce the very pressure you are trying to escape. They measure your worth through appearance, push you toward rigid routines, or keep you anchored in cycles of guilt. Others, however, become lifelines, places where your healing is supported, mirrored, and celebrated.

Accountability that nourishes you doesn't demand perfection. It offers encouragement, checks in with kindness, and invites reflection without judgment. It asks how you feel, not how you look. It holds space for progress, missteps, and everything in between.

Surround yourself with those who:

- Celebrate progress over perfection and honor the non-linear nature of healing

- Ask curious, not critical, questions that open space for honest conversation

- Share tools, stories, and reminders instead of shame, fear, or comparison

- Are living proof that health can be joyful, nourishing, and self-directed

You might find this through a trusted friend, an online group, a local circle, or a coaching relationship. The right community feels like a gentle container, not a tightrope.

Accountability should feel like support, not surveillance. It should nourish your confidence, not your fear. Find those who remind you who you are, not who you're supposed to be.

Protect the Energy You've Reclaimed

This work isn't just about skin. It's about the energy you've taken back from a system that drains you. Protect it.

- Say no to events, people, or habits that pull you out of alignment. Saying no is not selfish, it's self-respect. It's a way of creating boundaries that support your healing, not sabotage it. Each no is a yes to something more aligned.

- Say yes to what brings clarity, softness, and strength. Choose what replenishes you, not what performs for others.

- Be protective of your mornings, your mirror, and your mindset. Guard those first moments of the day as sacred. Let your reflection meet you with intention, not criticism.

You're not fragile. You're focused. And protecting your energy is how you stay strong.

In the final chapter, we'll come full circle. It's time to look at what beauty really is, how health and radiance intertwine, and why your story is part of something much bigger than your reflection.

CHAPTER 12:

What Beauty Really Is

Beauty was never meant to be chased. It was meant to be lived.

In every culture, every era, there has been a sense of reverence for the human form, not because of its flawlessness, but because of its vitality. Its *aliveness*. Somewhere along the way, modernity replaced reverence with resistance. But now, you're reclaiming it. You are learning to be your own hero.

So let's end where this began: in truth.

Beauty Is Not Youth

We've been sold the lie that beauty is synonymous with being young. That after a certain age, we fade. That visibility, worth, and sensuality belong only to the smooth-skinned. But youth is not the only season of beauty, it is only the first.

Age is not decay. It is deepening. It is accumulation. It is your body becoming a living library of everything you have experienced. Laugh lines are records of joy. Sunspots are souvenirs of summers well lived. Loose skin may speak of children born, of battles survived, of strength lived in the marrow and not just the muscle.

With time, your beauty becomes less about aesthetics and more about presence. People feel you before they see you. Your energy, your self-respect, your quiet confidence, these are magnetic in a way no product can replicate.

The older you get, the more radiant you become, if you let yourself be nourished instead of numbed. When you feed yourself well, sleep deeply, love with honesty, and move with purpose, you glow, not because you are trying to, but because you are alive in truth.

You were never meant to fear aging. You were meant to arrive fully into yourself.

Real beauty deepens. It does not disappear.

Beauty Is Not Compliance

You were not born to match an algorithm. You were not put here to contort yourself into symmetry or smoothness or sales conversions. You were not created to exist in a feed or to win approval through pixels. The beauty that *sells* is not the same as the beauty that *heals*.

Compliance teaches you to shrink, to edit, to question your instincts. It rewards sameness. But real beauty is sovereign. It does not ask for permission. It does not mold itself to trends. It is not obedient, it is original.

You don't owe the world polish. You owe yourself *presence*. The world has enough people trying to blend in. What we need are people who are grounded, awake, and unafraid to take up space in their most honest form.

You were born to be your own hero, not to mimic what sells, but to embody what's sacred. And that sacredness lives in your rawness, your rhythms, your realness.

Beauty Is Rhythm

True beauty lives in cycles. It pulses with hormones, breath, light, hunger, creation, destruction, and renewal. It's found in the flush after a walk, the softness after rest, the glow after real nourishment.

This rhythm is ancient. You are not meant to look the same every day. Your face shifts with your hormones, your energy changes with the seasons, and your body evolves across each life stage. There is wisdom in the wave, something that modern beauty culture has tried to flatten in the name of consistency.

When you align with your body's natural rhythm, through nourishing ancestral foods, deep sleep, gentle movement, and rest when needed, you become unmistakably magnetic. Your glow is not manufactured, it is cellular. It comes from the inside out.

The more you embrace your cycles instead of resisting them, the more grounded you become. The more you soften into your seasons, the more radiance you embody.

No filter can replicate that. No routine can force it. It's not about doing more. It's about syncing with what was always yours to begin with.

Beauty Is Connection

When you care for yourself in a way that's honest and ancestral, people feel it. You walk differently. Speak differently. Listen more. Compare less. Your energy becomes quieter, deeper, and more grounded. You begin to take up space without apology. This shift is not about becoming more attractive. It's about becoming more available, to yourself and to others.

This is how beauty becomes contagious, not through envy, but through *permission*. Real beauty invites connection. It inspires others not to replicate you, but to return to themselves.

When someone sees you living aligned, bare-faced and bright-eyed, it wakes something up in them. It whispers, "You can do this too." It reminds them that they can be their own hero too. And sometimes, seeing that lived example does more to heal than any product or plan ever could.

Connection is the medicine that modern beauty culture has forgotten. It is not curated. It is not filtered. It is felt. And it is what makes beauty meaningful.

Beauty Is Health, Embodied

Health is not just numbers. It's how you carry your body. It's your skin's tone, your voice's steadiness, your posture's grace. It is the ease in your joints and the clarity in your eyes. When your hormones are balanced, your gut is nourished, and your nervous system feels safe, you radiate a quiet kind of confidence, one that doesn't need to be announced.

This is not about chasing perfection. This is *biological radiance*. It is the outward glow of an inner harmony. A well-regulated nervous system shows up on your face. Stable blood sugar reflects in your mood. Liver function affects your complexion. Your skin is not separate from your internal systems. It is the messenger, the mirror.

This version of beauty does not come from products. It comes from habits. From honoring your hunger cues, sleeping deeply, moving consistently, and thinking thoughts that nourish rather than tear down. It comes from choosing foods that remember your ancestors and rejecting trends that disconnect you from your biology.

This kind of health-based beauty is available to you, regardless of age, shape, or skin type. And it is the kind that sustains. It doesn't ask you to perform, only to support what's already working for your body.

You are not broken. You are responding. And now, you're choosing to respond with care.

A Final Reflection

Look in the mirror today, not to fix, but to *see*.

That skin has healed cuts. That face has laughed and cried. Those eyes have witnessed grief, grace, and growth.

You are not a project. You are a presence.

And from this place of peace, you get to decide what beauty means now.

So let it be rooted. Let it be real. Let it be yours.

Be your own hero. You already are.

In the Appendix, you'll find tools to continue this journey: DIY recipes, resources, and a journal to help you track your progress, not just in skin, but in sovereignty.

APPENDIX:

Tools for the Journey

This is your companion section. Practical, grounded, and meant to be used. Healing isn't linear, but with the right tools, it becomes sustainable. These recipes, resources, and prompts are here to help you apply what you've read—day by day, with intention. Be your own hero.

DIY Ancestral Skincare Recipes

1. Whipped Tallow Balm

Ingredients:

- 1 cup grass-fed beef tallow (rendered and strained)
- 1/4 cup organic coconut oil
- Optional: 3–5 drops lavender or frankincense essential oil

Instructions:

1. Warm tallow gently in a double boiler until soft.
2. Mix in oil, stir well.
3. Let cool slightly, then whip with a hand mixer until fluffy.

4. Store in a glass jar. Use as moisturizer, balm, or makeup remover.

Be your own hero—nourish your skin with ingredients your great-grandmother would recognize.

---

2. Raw Honey Cleansing Mask

Ingredients:

- 1 tsp raw honey

- Optional: pinch of turmeric or cinnamon (patch test first)

Instructions:

1. Massage gently into damp skin.

2. Leave on for 10–15 minutes.

3. Rinse with warm water. Pat dry.

Let your skin heal with simplicity. Be your own hero.

---

3. Apple Cider Vinegar Toner

Ingredients:

- 1 part raw ACV
- 3 parts filtered water
- Optional: rose water or chamomile infusion

Instructions:

1. Combine in glass spray bottle.
2. Apply with cotton pad or spritz directly.
3. Store in a cool, dark place.

You don't need a lab—you need wisdom. Be your own hero.

---

4. Mineral Magnesium Deodorant Spray

Ingredients:

- 1/2 cup magnesium chloride flakes
- 1/2 cup distilled water

- Optional: 5–10 drops tea tree or eucalyptus essential oil

Instructions:

1. Dissolve flakes in warm water.

2. Let cool. Pour into glass spray bottle.

3. Apply to clean, dry underarms.

Support your body's natural detox process. Be your own hero.

Resources & Reading List

Organizations & Databases

- Environmental Working Group (EWG): ewg.org/skindeep

- Made Safe: madesafe.org

- Think Dirty App: Ingredient checker and product scanner

Books for Deeper Reading

- *Not Just a Pretty Face* by Stacy Malkan

- *The Beauty Myth* by Naomi Wolf

- *Hope in a Jar* by Kathy Peiss

- *In the FLO* by Alisa Vitti (hormone-health focused)

- *The Dirt Cure* by Maya Shetreat

Educate yourself, question everything, and always: be your own hero.

Reflection Journal Prompts

Use these prompts weekly or monthly to stay connected to your why, your body, and your growth:

- What was my relationship with beauty growing up?
- What messages about my skin/body do I still carry?
- What has shifted since starting my detox?
- Where do I still feel pressure to perform or perfect?
- How does my skin feel today?
- What does my skin need *from me*?
- What does beauty mean to me now?
- What will I teach the next generation about beauty?

Write your truth. Reclaim your story. Be your own hero.

Final Reminder

You don't need another protocol. You need presence. You need rhythm. You need reminders that you were never broken, only buried under a story that was never yours.

Come back to this appendix anytime you need to reconnect. You have what you need. You always did. Be your own hero.

References

- Fardouly, J., Diedrichs, P. C., Vartanian, L. R., & Halliwell, E. (2015). Social comparisons on social media: The impact of Facebook on young women's body image concerns and mood. *Body Image*, 13, 38–45.

- Henley, D. V., Lipson, N., Korach, K. S., & Bloch, C. A. (2007). Prepubertal gynecomastia linked to lavender and tea tree oils. *New England Journal of Medicine*, 356(5), 479–485.

- Perloff, R. M. (2014). Social media effects on young women's body image concerns: Theoretical perspectives and an agenda for research. *Sex Roles*, 71(11–12), 363–377.

- Tiggemann, M., & Slater, A. (2014). NetGirls: The Internet, Facebook, and body image concern in adolescent girls. *International Journal of Eating Disorders*, 47(6), 630–643.

- Environmental Working Group (EWG). (2022). *Skin Deep Database: The truth about your products*. Retrieved from https://www.ewg.org/skindeep/

- Tye, L. (1998). *The Father of Spin: Edward L. Bernays and the Birth of Public Relations*. Crown Publishing Group.

- Cash, T. F., & Smolak, L. (2011). *Body Image: A Handbook of Science, Practice, and Prevention*. Guilford Press.

- Dweck, C. S. (2008). *Mindset: The New Psychology of Success*. Ballantine Books.

- Groesz, L. M., Levine, M. P., & Murnen, S. K. (2002). The effect of experimental presentation of thin media images on body satisfaction: A meta-analytic review. *International Journal of Eating Disorders*, 31(1), 1–16.

- Cordain, L., Lindeberg, S., Hurtado, M., Hill, K., Eaton, S. B., & Brand-Miller, J. (2003). Acne vulgaris: A disease of Western civilization. *Archives of Dermatology*, 139(3), 354–359.

- Lio, P. A., & Katta, R. (2014). Diet and dermatology: The role of dietary intervention in skin disease. *Journal of Clinical and Aesthetic Dermatology*, 7(7), 46–51.

- Díaz-Ruiz, A., et al. (2018). Polyunsaturated fatty acid intake and skin aging: A review. *Nutrients*, 10(10), 1338.

- Ganguly, R., & Pierce, G. N. (2015). The toxicity of dietary oxidized cholesterol: A review. *Nutrition Reviews*, 73(9), 600–607.

- **Kiecolt-Glaser, J. K., et al.** (2010). Chronic stress and age-related increases in the proinflammatory cytokine IL-6. *PNAS*, 100(15), 9090–9095.

- **Russell, E., et al.** (2014). Hair cortisol as a biological marker of chronic stress: Current status, future directions and unanswered questions. *Psychoneuroendocrinology*, 38(5), 623–631.

- **Ober, C., Loisel, D. A., & Gilad, Y.** (2008). Sex-specific genetic architecture of human disease. *Nature Reviews Genetics*, 9(12), 911–922.

- **Turner, N. D., & Lloyd, S. K.** (2017). Association between red meat consumption and colon cancer: A systematic review of experimental results. *Journal of the American College of Nutrition*, 36(2), 106–115.

- **Price, W. A.** (1939). *Nutrition and Physical Degeneration*. Price-Pottenger Nutrition Foundation.

- **Thompson, J. K., & Stice, E.** (2001). Thin-ideal internalization: Mounting evidence for a new risk factor for body-image disturbance and eating pathology. *Current Directions in Psychological Science*, 10(5), 181–183.

Made in the USA
Monee, IL
25 May 2025